Ethics in General Practice

A practical handbook for personal development

Ann Orme-Smith

MA, MB BS, FRCGP

Full-time Principal in General Practice
Tadworth, Surrey

and

John Spicer

MB BS, MRCGP, DFFP, MA

General Practitioner
South Norwood, London
Course Organiser
Croydon VTS

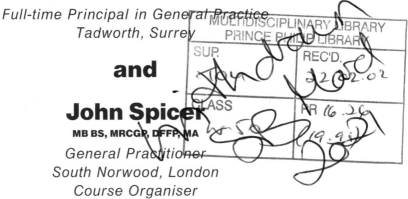

Foreword by

Professor Sean Hilton

Dean of Undergraduate Medicine
St George's Hospital Medical School
University of London

Radcliffe Medical Press Ltd
18 Marcham Road, Abingdon, Oxon OX14 1AA

British Library Cataloguing in Publication Data

A catalogue record for this book is available from the British Library.

ISBN 1 85775 328 3

Typeset by Aarontype Limited, Easton, Bristol
Printed and bound by TJ International Ltd, Padstow, Cornwall

Contents

Foreword

Anyone qualifying in medicine more than 10 years ago will have needed to acquire their knowledge and learning about medical ethics 'on the job' in postgraduate practice. Although undergraduate medical courses now, rightly, give much greater grounding in medical ethics, the subject area is an enormous one. This book is by Ann Orme-Smith and John Spicer, two experienced general practitioners with considerable combined experience in vocational training and postgraduate education for general practice. It provides thoughtful and very relevant reading for all those working in general practice in challenging times of societal and organisational change.

The opening chapters deal with the application of moral theories and the basic principles of ethics, and underline our need for ethically-based practice as well as evidence-based medicine. The two are not mutually exclusive, and we need both in order to practise modern medicine humanely and effectively.

A series of chapters on key issues such as confidentiality, preventive medicine, mental health problems, consent, infertility, paediatrics, and end of life issues are covered helpfully, in ways that relate the law as it stands currently to the relevant ethical aspects and principles. The text is richly illustrated with common clinical scenarios that will be easily recognised by all practising clinicians, and the whole book is strongly grounded in general practice.

The final chapter demonstrates why this book is so important. The changes to the NHS in the UK, and in clinical practice, are examined for the challenges they will pose for general practitioners in the coming years.

Ethics in General Practice is dedicated to John Lasserson, and is a fitting tribute to a highly ethical practitioner, whose untimely death robbed Orme-Smith and Spicer of a third co-author for this fine book.

Professor Sean Hilton
General Practitioner
Dean of Undergraduate Medicine
St George's Hospital Medical School, University of London
February 2001

Preface

A working understanding of medical ethics is becoming ever more important to all practising doctors, not least the general practitioner. The high-profile ethical problems such as cloning and genetic engineering that exercise the public mind tend not to be particularly relevant to GPs and their patients. There are, however, many everyday ethical issues which present, often unexpectedly, to the GP and which can seem impossible to resolve.

This book introduces some of these important issues, using examples, and encourages a deeper exploration than the reader may previously have been able to accomplish. Legal aspects are included where they are relevant to the main topic in each chapter. We have included speculation on the future, being well aware of the probable expansion in this area.

The text is designed primarily for GPs in training, at whatever stage. It is explanatory rather than exploratory. Experienced GPs who wish to expand their ethical understanding will find this a useful introductory text, and perhaps a spur to further interest. Any health professional or lay person with a particular interest in primary care may also find the text useful.

Case histories are named in alphabetical order within each chapter and are drawn mainly from the experience of the authors. Often these cases are composite. No connection to identifiable persons is intended nor should any be made. Where reference is made to a GP as 'him' or 'her' it is purely random.

References are used to amplify the text, note a journal citation or reference a legal case. Many are clinical, and refer to leading medical journals that are easily accessed. All bear further reading.

Ethical points are repeated in different chapters and are cross-referenced. This is intentional: the book is constructed so that the content of each chapter stands on its own.

Different chapters will reveal contrasts in style and reasoning. Sometimes potential 'answers' are revealed and sometimes not, according to the subject under discussion. All chapters have pointers to further thought or analysis that the reader might find of benefit.

Ann Orme-Smith
John Spicer
February 2001

Acknowledgements

We thank all those friends, GP colleagues and registrars who have given us useful comments on the preparation of the text, in particular Eileen Allan, Deborah Bowman, Mary Clarke, Richard Howarth, Ann King, Charlotte Knight, Helen Lees and Jeremy Shindler, but especially our partners at home, David and Ley.

CHAPTER ONE

Learning about ethics: why is it important?

Learning about ethics has only recently been recognised as being of high priority in medical training: some of our current population of doctors have sworn the Hippocratic Oath, but most have not. Some had exposure to moral and ethical thinking in medical school, but most did not. Some doctors studied humanities or other non-scientific disciplines before medicine, but most did not. The situation is changing, and the newer generations of doctors will have greater time given as undergraduates to ethical and legal matters.[1] These important subjects are now part of the core undergraduate curriculum.[2]

Why is it important to study such an ephemeral subject as ethics, where it could be said that discussion and debate lead nowhere and there is no one unequivocal ethical solution to a problem? For example, where an ethics module is included within the medical curriculum, how could such an expenditure of time and resources be justified? There are some cogent arguments against such a proposal. It could be said that there are no universally applicable rules in ethics, that it is a mish-mash of opinions. In any given situation, there may be so many conflicting issues that decision making would be made too complicated if we took all of them into consideration. Introducing ideas of equality and autonomy, which then pull in opposite directions, would make it impossible to accommodate everyone's interests. It sounds good in theory, but is likely to be time-consuming in practice. We could argue that there is nothing wrong with a pragmatic system governed by the use of experience, intuition and common sense.

The bulk of medical teaching trains doctors to work according to evidence-based clinical protocols for diagnosis and treatment. Introducing an ethical dimension into everyday medical practice requires them to look at their work from another perspective.[3] Apart from the educational advantage of expanding the boundaries of medical training, there is the probable beneficial impact on patient care. There might be a better chance of recognising the full range of issues in any given situation that would promote a wider choice of options for action. Insight and awareness of the deep-seated attitudes and prejudices that influence decisions increases the likelihood of flexibility of approach rather than emotional entrenchment. This could provide impartiality with the probability of better outcomes for the patient. Credibility may be strengthened, patient care improved, and well-reasoned decisions can be openly defended.

In the past, when paternalism reigned, with doctors making decisions on behalf of their patients, supposedly having their best interests in mind and following Hippocratic guidance of beneficence and non-maleficence, the ethical content of patient care could be reduced to the minimum. The application of philosophical theory and the existence of conflicting attitudes had little part to play; there needed to be a considerable element of trust in the medical profession by patients and the public. Attitudes have changed, paternalism is replaced by partnership where patients' autonomy is recognised. People are in general better informed about healthcare and have a better understanding of the standards they can expect. Trust remains a crucial component of the doctor–patient relationship but it is based on a fuller mutual understanding and on a more equal footing than prevailed in the past.

It would be a mistake to make too many assumptions about people's understanding. For many the doctor is the one with the expertise and the answers to their problems and, as such, is invested with a certain amount of power in the relationship. It is easy for the doctor to accept this role and make most decisions on his patient's behalf. Advances in medicine make it difficult to provide information to patients in an accessible form; it could be said that a little knowledge would provoke more anxiety than none at all. When should information be given, how much, and can it be guaranteed that the patient has understood?

Virtually all GP consultations have an ethical dimension, which may be more or less obvious. Ultimately, the patient is better served by a GP who considers this dimension as an integral part of each interaction with a patient.

What is meant by 'medical ethics'?

Ethics has been defined as:

> the philosophical study of the moral value of human conduct and of the rules and principles that ought to govern it; . . . a code of behaviour considered correct especially that of a particular group, profession or individual.[4]

We could say that in order to know how to behave in an ethical manner we need to use a background of moral philosophy from which we deduce certain principles on which we ought to act. This is in contrast to the opinion that we can organise our professional behaviour using pre-existing human qualities that tell us by instinct how to make the right decisions, or by so-called professional self-regulation.

When we approach the subject of medical ethics we are in the arena of deciding what is the *right* course of action as opposed to *wrong*. For example, is it right or wrong to give a certain treatment, to withdraw it, to choose one treatment rather than another, or to look for disease before evaluating symptoms? In this, medicine is no different from any other profession: moral choices will arise for consideration and will need to be weighed in the balance.

Yet it is because healthcare in our society is of fundamental importance that the actions of healthcare professionals and choices made by patients are exposed to critical assessment. Using the words 'right' and 'wrong' in this context might suggest that clear cut answers can be found by a process of analysis. Is this so?

Consider the following case.

Alan is 43 and drinks heavily. His GP has known him and his family over many years. He is being prosecuted by the police for driving with an illegal quantity of alcohol in his body. He comes to see his GP for help, saying his asthma prevented him blowing properly into the alcometer used by the police.

It is not difficult to see that there are many conflicting pressures here. The GP will have a duty to do the best for Alan and his family, but will also be conscious of a duty to assist the law in process, as exemplified by the police prosecution. She will be aware of the needs of confidentiality when making reports to court, but might also feel that Alan should 'get his deserts' as an ordinary citizen too. She might worry over Alan's family, who will be the poorer when he loses his job that depends on his ability to drive. An understanding of medical ethics will help Alan's GP to find the best course of action and to answer the question: what ought to be done?

Ethics, morals and the law

The words *ethical* and *moral* are used frequently in this book. Both refer to *behaviour* – good and bad, right and wrong. In moral terms, what is the right decision going to be? This might seem a daunting task, as Alan's GP's problem exemplifies. However, we do have sources of guidance. One obvious one is the law, which is often poorly understood by doctors but can sometimes be helpful.

> Betty is a cantankerous lady who constantly finds fault with what members of the primary healthcare team try to do to help her. She has multiple physical problems that the GP, community nurses and physiotherapists grapple with as best they can. Their best never seems to be good enough. One day she comes to see the doctor and asks for copies of all her computer records over the last year. She won't say why.

The GP is ambivalent about this unexplained request, unsure as to whether she ought to comply. What is she to do?

The answer is straightforward if uncomfortable. Statute law is uncompromising[5] and the GP must provide Betty with the records, within certain clearly defined limits (*see* also Chapter 3).[6] Is there an ethical basis for this law? The relevant statutes here are an expression of *autonomy*, the principle that exemplifies the fact that patients ought to have dominion over their own affairs, including information held by doctors about them. This principle disallows paternalistic behaviour by doctors, and says that people should be agents of their own destiny.

It is arguably the most important principle in medical ethics today, and we will be addressing it in greater detail in succeeding chapters. Much of our law in this country, including these statutes, is codifying the moral principle of autonomy. It converts what we take, morally, as being a *right* action into an *obligatory* one, with the force of law. It is important to remember that for most of the time doctors will not have the law to instruct them in non-clinical decision making, as with the problem posed to Alan's GP.

Moral theories

Man has always struggled with distinguishing 'right' decisions from those that are 'wrong'. The discipline of moral philosophy is founded on this struggle and its content feeds modern considerations of medical ethics.

Ethics, historically, is a branch of philosophy, the study of beliefs and values. Philosophy deals mostly in theory, though interestingly enough, in an article praising applied philosophy, one author has suggested that the true philosophers of today reside in hospitals and laboratories (to which we could add GP surgeries).[7]

We will be considering these four main moral theories in this book:

- virtue
- duty
- utility
- rights

which are four different ways of answering the question 'What is the right thing to do?'

Like all theories, moral theories are only speculative. They cannot be disproved or proved, and in the medical context they represent a way of analysing particular problems. For those with a scientific background, such as most doctors, this does not come naturally.

Generally, scientists prefer to ascribe truth to a proposition that can be proved objectively rather than to a speculative one.

Recent years have seen a trend towards justifying doctors' actions in diagnosis or treatment on evidential grounds – evidence-based practice. Whilst this is laudable, it is a different process from moral reasoning which deals in uncertainties and logical analysis.

The moral theories listed above are broad strands of thought in moral philosophy and they underpin most modern-day medical ethics, even if they have ancient roots. Let us have a closer look at them.

Virtue ethics can be traced back to Aristotle. The theory is that people with certain intrinsic good character traits make good decisions, and we should aspire to exhibit such qualities. For the soldier, that might be bravery or fortitude, for the parson, truthfulness and temperance. It is arguable what virtues a modern healthcare professional should have: perhaps determination, consistency and a sense of humanity. Modern moral philosophers have reawakened interest in virtue ethics and there are rich sources of further reading for the interested GP.[8,9]

That there should be **duties** in medical practice may seem obvious, but one needs to ask why that should be so. This moral theory holds that we have obligations to each other based upon respect for one another's person. The theory is associated mainly with the German philosopher, Kant, who formulated what he described as the *categorical imperative*, defining our duty to each other as human beings. One version of this is that people should always be regarded and treated as 'ends' rather than 'means', as a measure of respect.

For example, a doctor with profound objections to abortion may hold that respect for the person begins at conception, and that confers a duty upon him not to interfere with that person by engineering its destruction in any way. The Roman Catholic Church holds such a view, and this guides and instructs most Catholic doctors. It is one aspect of a moral principle known as the *sanctity of life*; clearly, this can also be held from a secular perspective.

More recently the theory of **utility** has been expounded by Jeremy Bentham and John Stuart Mill, and represents a dramatic advance. Utility states that the rightness and wrongness of actions are determined only by their consequences. If an action produces the greatest good for the greatest number it is, by definition, the right action.

Consider organ donation. It is powerfully argued that the UK should move to a system of 'opting out': access to organs after death by transplant teams should be allowed automatically unless the individual has 'opted out' by expressing a wish that their organs are not used in this way. This serves the greater good for all. Recipient patients benefit more because more organs would be available to keep them alive, and nobody suffers because the donors are dead anyway. Respect for the dead or their relatives is all that is infringed.

If benefits and disadvantages of this system are weighed up, opting out would be favoured. In spite of this many would find it difficult to accept, but the *utilitarian* would have no problem: the greatest good for the greatest number is served.[10] GPs make many such decisions in the modern-day cost-limited NHS, where the theory of utility informs decision making.[11]

The theory of **rights** is a more modern notion. The right to medical care is expressed often and in many different ways; this right today governs a great deal of access to medical care. For example, everyone has a *right* to the services of a GP, enshrined in law by the National Health Service Act and the Terms and Conditions of Service that govern the GP service.[12]

Applying moral theories

One of the difficulties with medical ethics is the attachment of the word 'medical', almost as if the observance and understanding of ethics in the practice of medicine is somehow different, separate, from the rest of human morality. In this book we suggest that every doctor–patient interaction has an ethical dimension, which may be explored beneficially from a general moral viewpoint rather than a more restricted medical perspective. Although the examples that are used will come from everyday general practice experience their discussion ought not to be exclusively medical.

Questioning and discussion of the broader issues of ethics helps towards the clearer understanding of the various ways through some of the complex dilemmas that appear daily in the small world of general practice. For example, in the consulting room with a patient, if we regard the interchange and its outcome as confined within a pure medical ethical model, much of the patient's being is excluded. The medical ethics may be straightforward and clear, governed by the concept of 'good medical practice'; it may be that the ethical challenge arises at a deeper, more complex level when the patient is regarded, not merely as a purveyor of a disease process, but as a person.

Ethical interest lies in conflict and its resolution, and intuition is an element not to be ignored. Unfortunately, medical training tends to impress on the student the importance of 'evidence-based medicine' where intuitive responses have no place. Perhaps the moral response to many of the conflicts that a GP will see in everyday practice would be better defined if the GP considered them not only as a doctor but as a morally intuitive human being.

We can attempt to solve some of the main ethical dilemmas in general practice by referring to the various philosophical arguments. Bentham and Mill's *utilitarian* theory – the greatest happiness concept – could form the basis of resource allocation. In dispensing defined resources in order to achieve maximum overall benefit, who gets what treatment, how much, and when? What will the *consequences* be – how much benefit will there be for the general population, immediately and in the long term? But in conflict with this arrangement, there is Kant and his categorical imperative. Each man is to be treated as a person in his own right, never as a means to an end.

Thus *rights-based* ethical decisions, founded on respect for others as individuals, take place in the consulting room, with regard to that particular patient whose rights are paramount. The doctor's integrity and self-respect will depend very much on his sense of his own moral *virtue*; he will be reluctant to be swayed towards making decisions which are in conflict with his intuitive sense of moral right. If others around him regard him as a 'good' person, whose actions and expressed attitudes coincide with Aristotle's virtuous man, he will attract respect and support from his fellows.

These are the traditional approaches to ethics from the perspective of moral philosophy; all have something to contribute to the resolution of the medico-moral problems that doctors have to face.

Four ethical principles

Another perspective of more recent provenance is shown below. This consists of a list of irreducible principles that ought to govern all ethical decision making in clinical practice. They were suggested by two American ethicists, Beauchamp and Childress,[13] and later developed by Gillon, a GP and medical ethicist:[14]

- autonomy
- beneficence
- non-maleficence
- justice.

It is argued that consideration of these *prima facie* principles aids the debate of any ethical problem confronting a healthcare worker. It is important to remember that the application of ethical principles will not invariably lead to the resolution of such problems. Let us have a closer look at them.

Autonomy has been touched on already: the capacity of people to make their own decisions. We might say that a fully autonomous decision would require knowledge of all the facts, and should be free and uncoerced.

Colin has three children and comes to the practice to see the nurse one evening. He asks about having a vasectomy, saying: 'My wife sent me down for the snip, but I'm worried, doesn't it give you cancer sometimes or make you need Viagra ....'.

The nurse talks about the complications of vasectomy and allays his fears, but she still thinks he is doing his wife's bidding. She is unsure whether to refer him.

It might seem that autonomy is always limited, since we can never be in possession of all the facts, but the nurse here has facilitated an autonomous choice more clearly than before. She still has reservations about the consultation: has Colin's autonomy been undermined by his wife's coercion? Further counselling will no doubt be called for.

Non-maleficence is the principle that we should do no harm. Most remember the Latin maxim *'primum non nocere'* – 'firstly do no harm', said to be an all-embracing principle for doctors.

Doris had withdrawn from taking the appetite suppressants that she had been addicted to for many years. Over months this had required much support from the team at the practice. Recently she had become obese again and very tired. She asked if she could have only a short course of them again 'to make me feel better'. Her GP considered her request carefully but refused, suggesting other ways of handling the problem.

This doctor must have been thinking of the harm that a new prescription could do to Doris, and demurred, not wanting to expose her to the risk of addiction or to other drug side effects. It could be argued that despite her wish (or autonomous decision) the doctor allowed the principle of non-maleficence to dominate.

The doctor here acted with **beneficence** by suggesting other ways of handling her problem. Perhaps he arranged further work with her, or did some tests, but at all events followed a course of management directed to her best interests, as he saw them. We will be looking at this term 'best interests' in more detail later. It has a more complex legal meaning than is apparent at first sight.

Justice is a population-based principle. The interpretation we shall be using is that of *distributive* justice, to differentiate it from the better known interpretation of *retributive* justice, the process that involves the criminal law in punishment. Under this principle, justice is created and fostered by those in control – governments, health authorities, primary care groups – when they allocate funds with fairness according to need. There are many ways this might be done, and increasingly primary healthcare teams are involved in this decision making.

Ed is an alcoholic in end stage liver disease. His drinking is now under control after many years of abuse. He has used many different NHS resources to get to where he is. He is being considered for a liver transplant, but his health authority (HA) have decided not to provide the funds. Evidence seems to suggest alcoholics in end stage liver disease do less well after operation than other patients. Ed asks his GP to help in changing their view so that he can go for surgery.

Traditionally, resource allocation decisions are not made by those caring directly for patients. This is changing, and increasingly GPs have to face patients who are suffering the results of resource decisions. This GP might sit on an advisory board to the HA and be in a quandary. If the HA is right and the evidence is as they say, is their decision just? It could be argued that the causation of the liver disease is immaterial and the surgeons must accept the comparative postoperative success rates in the name of equality of access. Perhaps there are other factors relevant to Ed: whether he has a family to support, or how long he has been abstinent. Should Ed have a right to surgery based upon his NHS contributions in taxation anyway? We pose these questions as illustrative of the problems that an ethical understanding might resolve.

These are some of the moral theories that have constituted ethical thinking over the centuries, from which doctors and many health professionals take their lead. There may be no easy answers in medical ethics, and yet clearly defined ethical principles can give direction. In the words of a fictional character faced with a moral dilemma:

> He said: 'But it wouldn't be playing the game!' A long time afterwards he said 'Damn all principles!' And then: 'But one has to keep going ... Principles are like the skeleton map of a country – you know whether you're going east or north.'[15]

References and notes

1 Consensus statement by teachers of medical ethics and law in UK medical schools (1998) Teaching medical ethics and law within medical education: a model for the UK core curriculum. *J Med Ethics.* **24**: 188–92.

2 Doyal L and Gillon R (1998) Medical ethics and law as a core subject in medical education. *BMJ.* **316**: 1623–4.

3 'There is a paucity of research into the ethical concerns of general practice'. Rogers WA (1997) A systematic review of empirical research into ethics in general practice. *BJ Gen Pract.* **47**: 733–7.

4 *Collins English Dictionary* (1994) HarperCollins, Glasgow.

5 The medical defence organisations will give legal advice on request.

6 To summarise the provisions of the Data Protection Acts 1994 and 1998, the Access to Medical Reports Act 1988 and the Access to Health Records

Act 1990: a patient may see and correct inaccuracies in any record from 1 Nov 91 unless serious harm to the patient's physical or mental health might occur by such a disclosure.

7 Cohen M (1998) Philosophical Notes. *Independent* 13 September 1998, p. 11.
8 Toon P (1999) *Towards a Philosophy of General Practice: a study of the virtuous practitioner* (Occasional Paper 78). RCGP, London.
9 McIntyre A (1981) *After Virtue.* Duckworth, London.
10 One author has described a hypothetical human lottery. Each citizen has a unique lottery number. A need for organs would initiate the random selection of a number by computer. That citizen would then provide organs for the needy patients. Greater numbers would survive: a truly utilitarian argument. Harris J (1986) The Survival Lottery. In: P Singer (ed.) *Applied Ethics.* Oxford University Press, Oxford.
11 The GP's interest in such decisions has become necessary with the emergence of direct GP involvement via primary care groups (PCGs).
12 Sometimes medical care can infringe a right: when a patient is confined under the Mental Health Act for good clinical reasons, their right to liberty is removed, albeit temporarily.
13 Beauchamp TL and Childress JF (1994) *Principles of Medical Ethics* (4e). Oxford University Press, Oxford.
14 Gillon R (1994) Four principles plus scope. *BMJ.* **309**: 184–8.
15 Ford Madox Ford (1997) *Parade's End.* Carcanet Press, Manchester, p. 144.

CHAPTER TWO

Professional duties: 'Trust me, I'm a doctor'

Summary

This chapter demonstrates the importance of integrating ethical reasoning into the everyday work of the GP under the following headings:

- Formal duties – ability and judgement
- Accountability and competence – the General Medical Council
- Humanity and beneficence – compassion
- Consent to treatment – implied and explicit
- Protecting patients
- Special relationships
- The public view
- Paternalism power and conflict – 'hard cases'.

he said I'm real sorry he said I wish I had some other kind of news
to give you
I said Amen and he said something else
I didn't catch and not knowing what else to do
and not wanting him to have to repeat it
and me to have to fully digest it

*I just looked at him for a minute and he looked back and it
was then
I jumped up and shook hands with this man who'd just given me
something that no one else on earth had ever given me
I may even have thanked him habit being so strong.*[1]

Introduction

In his poem, Raymond Carver is describing his memory of the
interchange he had with his doctor, who was giving him some bad
news.[1] The words give an illuminating insight into the fundamental relationship between doctor and patient. The doctor's position is one of power; he has information about his patient's illness
that he may choose to share with that patient – or not. In the
event, he gives the bad news and his patient thanks him for it, out
of habit. And yet the trust that the patient has in his doctor, to tell
him the truth – truth tempered by compassion – is matched by the
doctor's own sense of moral duty to his patient. It is this delicate
balance which underlies the many facets of the doctor's professional duty.

The medical training that is currently provided in this country is
aimed in the most part at producing a basic level of competence
in the newly qualified doctor. This competence will be grounded in
scientific knowledge of human physiology, anatomy, presentation of
symptoms and diagnosis of disease. The evidence base of diagnosis
and treatment is continually expanding, as is the range of specialisa-
tion in medicine. The doctor in training in the future cannot be
expected to have a full working knowledge of every advance that is
made; he will be ever more aware of how much he does not know.
Where appropriate, he will need to be prepared to confess ignorance
rather than pretend to be the all-knowing expert.

In this chapter we widen the view of the doctor as a scientific
expert, and look at the general practitioners' (GP) moral and ethical
place in society. This will necessarily entail speculation of the
patient's expectations of doctors as a professional group, and of his
own doctor in particular.

Formal duties

Ethical principles of beneficence and non-maleficence

> It really is of importance, not only what men do, but also what manner of men they are that do it. Among the works of man, which human life is rightly employed in perfecting and beautifying, the first in importance surely is man himself.[2]

Under this heading we consider the ethical elements of good medical practice (GMP). Every doctor is now expected to practise to a minimum standard and to keep up to date, and soon will need to demonstrate competence under the system of revalidation (*see* below).[3] Continuing professional development (CPD) and clinical governance form part of this process.

The relationship between a doctor and patient depends on trust, which is defined as 'reliance on and confidence in the truth, worth, reliability, etc., of a person or thing'.[4] Anything that threatens that trust is potentially damaging to the relationship, and the patient could be harmed as a result.

The recent proliferation of 'bad doctor'cases, substantially reported in the media, poses just such a threat. The reporting is not the issue: it is important that this happens, and that the public is properly informed of these cases. The problems are rarely due to intentional transgressions of the relevant section of the Hippocratic Oath: 'I will follow that system of regimen which, according to my ability and judgement, I consider for the benefit of my patients, and abstain from whatever is deleterious and mischievous' (*see* Appendix 1). In other words, 'I will pursue a course of beneficence, and refrain from maleficence.' True maleficence, fortunately, is very rare: the most recent case concerned a GP.[5]

More often, it is the *ability* and *judgement* of the doctor that has been seriously questioned. The patient's trust is based on these aspects of care – the intrinsic worth of the doctor's professional values – together with the expectation that the doctor will be truthful.

Therefore the doctor has a duty to respond to this trust by ensuring that he maintains acceptable standards of clinical competence and decision making. As is stated by the General Medical Council, 'the public has a right to expect considerate and competent medical attention from doctors. And doctors have a duty to maintain a good standard of professional work.'[6]

Accountability and competence

Ethical principle of justice

The medical profession is regulated by the General Medical Council (GMC). This is a body with 104 members, the majority of whom are fully registered doctors. The preponderance of medical members has occasioned criticism of the continuing system of 'self-regulation' of the medical profession. The publicity surrounding recent high-profile cases of serious professional misconduct has led to accusations of undue delay on the part of the GMC in dealing with the doctors under scrutiny. Should not the public be protected against the dangers of malpractice at the earliest possible stage?

On the other hand, doctors are vulnerable to unfounded complaints and justice demands that each one accused be given a fair hearing once all the evidence has been collected. A complaint to the GMC is a serious matter, and if proven, could cost the doctor his or her livelihood. The whole procedure takes time and meanwhile, the doctor continues to see patients. Some feel that the workings of the GMC, with its preponderance of medical members, are organised in a way that results in part in the medical profession 'protecting its own'. There is an inherent conflict between the protection of patients from harm and the protection of doctors from false accusations; a balance needs to be struck which is ethically sound.

The GMC was established first under the Medical Act 1858 on the recommendation of the recently formed British Medical Association. The Medical Act stated that 'it is expedient that persons requiring medical aid should be able to distinguish qualified from unqualified practitioners'.

The GMC's role has developed since 1858, and it now has three main functions (see Chapter 6 for a full description of the role of the GMC):[7]

1 to maintain a register of fully qualified doctors
2 to administer disciplinary sanctions to doctors found unfit to practise[8]
3 to issue guidance on medical ethics and standards of conduct expected of doctors.[9]

The GMC is currently extending its regulatory function in the area of continuing professional competence. The revalidation programme is designed to assess the work of every registered doctor according to the requirements of his or her specialty. If it functions well, poor performance will be identified and rectified before harm comes to patients. The rationale for this is to *confirm* to patients and the public a doctor's *current* fitness to practise. It also has a formative function in encouraging doctors to maintain and improve standards of patient care.

There is the moral duty for every doctor to seek help if he or she is physically or mentally sick, and to stop practising until fit enough to continue. Patients can be put at risk if their doctor's good judgement is threatened by his own ill-health. In particular, alcohol or drugs are used to combat stress by doctors as much as they are by their patients and their use or abuse could affect adversely the quality of patient care. Yet drug and alcohol abuse carries a stigma. Accepting advice to seek help for such a problem can be difficult: it means that the doctor has to admit openly that it exists.

The behaviour of colleagues sometimes causes concern. 'Whistle blowing' on another doctor, whether for doubtful clinical competence, poor communication skills, suspicion of substance abuse, or any other sign of poor performance and possible risk to patients, can be extremely difficult to contemplate. Very often the first clue to the existence of a problem is only a vague supposition, and may be unsubstantiated. There is no way of telling how many others have noticed a similar problem, and are constrained from taking action.

There are particular problems for those working in hospital practice. The hierarchical system and the reliance on good references for the next job are said to be factors restraining the potential whistle blower.[10] These factors do not apply in general practice to any great extent, although it is possible for the GP registrar to feel similar restraints in the training practice.

The duty of any doctor to act in these difficult circumstances is clear in the GMC ethical guidance:

You must protect patients when you believe that a doctor's or other colleague's health, conduct or performance is a threat to them. Before taking action, you should do your best to find out the facts. Then, if necessary, you must follow your employer's procedures or tell an appropriate person from the employing authorities, such as the director of public health, medical director, nursing director or chief executive, or an officer of your local medical committee,[11] or a regulatory body. Your comments about colleagues must be honest. If you are not sure what to do, ask an experienced colleague or contact the GMC for advice. The safety of patients must come first at all times.[12]

GPs tend to work in a more independent way than those in hospital practice. Sometimes they work in isolation and do not have much contact with their GP colleagues; there may be little opportunity for observation of work patterns that are out of the ordinary. A sick GP may continue to work long after he ought to have stopped; fear of 'letting the practice down' or admitting a weakness constrain many from consulting their own GP. The illusion that 'doctors are never ill' still pervades the profession.

A problem may be evident to an employee in the GP practice, for example, the practice nurse or the GP registrar, long before other colleagues or partners. Hints of unsatisfactory variations from normal practice may also come from patients.

Nancy had a stroke years ago and has gradually deteriorated since then. She is in a wheelchair and never goes out. Her daughter Olive lives with her and is her only carer. Nancy has become very chesty again. Tonight Olive has asked for a visit from you, the GP on call for the local out-of-hours co-operative. Olive seems relieved to see you rather than anyone else. She tells you that last week one of the other GPs in the co-op was very rude to her mother. In his haste he tore her night-dress when examining her chest, and smelt strongly of drink. This GP is one of your colleagues in the neighbouring practice.

The story is one of unacceptable behaviour on the part of a GP. There is no reason to doubt its veracity – it is unusual for people to fabricate such stories. Is Olive to be believed? How serious is the accusation and how ought the visiting GP to react? If the report is true, is this acceptable behaviour in another GP who has the clinical responsibility for a large number of patients in the on-call rota system for the co-op? This number includes those on your practice list and that of your partners.

> The GP in question is well respected locally. You have not heard anything else about him that would support Olive's story. Do you take any action, and if so, what do you do?

It is important to recognise the ethical dimension of this problem. On the one hand, there is a duty to protect patients from possible harm, yet on the other, justice dictates that the doctor is able to answer any accusation made against him. Olive does not appear to have made an accusation, but her remarks are significant enough to cause concern. Consideration of the ethics involved will contribute to a resolution of the conflict.

Humanity and beneficence

The maintenance of good professional standards is a *basic* responsibility of every doctor; this responsibility involves not only medical competence, but consideration for the patient.[6]

The medical profession is regarded as a 'caring profession'. By this, we mean that as well as being one of the so-called 'learned' professions, together with law and theology, it requires its members to show compassion – the desire to relieve distress. Medicine is also a scientific discipline, where clinical expertise is reliant on a firm base of evidence and demonstrable practical skills. It would be ethically wrong to use an untried treatment, or to perform a clinical procedure unsupervised the first time.[13]

If medicine was only a science, a patient might be regarded only as a mechanical object, illness as a malfunction of the machine, and the doctor as a technician who knows how to correct the malfunction. Clearly this is far from the truth; medicine as an art acknowledges the patient as a human being, and the practice of medicine requires humanity on the part of the doctor.[14]

Pam has had a dry cough for some weeks, and has tried home remedies to no avail, indeed, it seems to be getting worse, and she is rather breathless. You know that she looks after her disabled husband who is registered blind. She had a mastectomy for breast cancer two years ago, and was depressed for some time afterwards, worrying about her husband. Who would look after him if she died?

She missed her last hospital check-up a month ago. When you examine her, her chest appears clear today. She is very pleased at this news.

Pam may only be suffering from a mild but persistent viral infection, and can be offered reassurance and symptomatic relief. More serious is the possibility of secondaries from her breast cancer, and maybe an effusion that you have not managed to detect.

You tell Pam that she needs to have a chest X-ray. She asks you why this is necessary. How much do you tell her of your concerns?

As soon as a person enters the surgery, he or she becomes a 'patient' – to the doctor, to the receptionist, to others in the practice. This does not, and should not, mean that the patient has ceased to be a person, with desires and fears that may not be expressed very clearly. Pam's GP can only guess at Pam's feelings about her cancer, her caring role at home, and the future. Sensitive exploration of these areas with Pam may give some helpful insight, but this is by no means certain.

Respecting Pam's autonomy by explaining the true reason for the X-ray – the need to exclude spread of her cancer – confronts Pam with the next question: if it has spread, what then? She may have recovered from her fears two years ago only to have them rekindled today. The GP may interpret her failure to attend her last hospital appointment as a reluctance to be reminded of the mastectomy and the reason for it. Is it kinder to give a non-committal reply? After all, the GP's fears may be totally unfounded, and Pam will have been spared uncertainty and possible anguish; yet if the X-ray confirms the presence of secondaries, how will Pam's trust in her GP to respect her autonomy and tell her the truth be affected?

It may be that compassion means making some difficult decisions. The fear of giving a person pain conflicts with the desire to be truthful at all times.

For those who provide care to cancer patients, the challenge is finding a way of providing information that is appropriate to patients who may benefit from knowing something about their illness and its treatment but may not wish to know everything about it at all times.[15]

Consent to treatment

Ethical principle of autonomy, or self-determination

No doctor ought to presume to treat a patient, who is competent to make his or her own decisions, without consent. Indeed to do so would be to run the risk of an action for battery: unlawful touching (*see* Chapters 6 and 8 for consent to treatment of incompetent children and adults). The law reflects the ethical principle of autonomy, and firmly supports patients' rights in this respect.

Valid consent depends on:

- competence to understand the full implications of the treatment
- adequate information on the nature of the treatment to be agreed
- voluntariness – lack of coercion or undue influence from others.

These criteria for valid consent demand a considerable ethical commitment by the doctor. Simple matters can be quickly and easily explained to the patient of reasonable intelligence. More complicated matters will take more time and effort on the part of the doctor in attempting to explain them to a patient with communication difficulties due to language, deafness or intellectual capability.[16]

Implied consent

Many of the patients that a GP sees during surgery sessions are assumed to have implied consent by their very presence in the consulting room. Courtesy will direct the GP to ask the patient for consent before starting an examination, but he may not consider expanding on the reason for the examination. It is often obvious: the patient with a cough or sore throat is likely to expect an examination of the chest or pharynx.

Only if the examination were not obviously relevant to the presenting symptom would the patient expect an explanation. Without an explanation the teenage girl with a sore throat may not understand the necessity for her GP to take some blood and examine her axillae and upper abdomen as well as her throat. She will need to understand that her GP wishes to test her blood for signs of glandular fever and look for enlarged glands and spleen. He will also have to use words she can understand rather than 'lymphadenopathy' and 'splenomegaly'.

Explicit consent

Much of the patient care carried out in the GP practice is with the patient's implied consent; it relies on the patient's trust that the GP will act in a way that the patient expects. If the GP asks the patient to roll up a sleeve and puts on a sphygmomanometer cuff, the patient no doubt expects the GP to take his blood pressure. He will not expect a venepuncture unless the GP has first explained what is about to happen before approaching his arm with a needle: some people with a needle phobia would refuse consent immediately. The GP will also need to inform the patient of the reason for the test, and exactly what will be included. There are some tests that give significant information that the patient may not wish to deal with unless adequately informed and prepared. HIV testing is an obvious example; it is customary to counsel patients carefully to ensure they understand the implications of the test before carrying this out.

You receive a package containing the equipment to take a sample of blood for DNA testing of Richard. He and his wife have been patients of yours for some years. They have no children. You have seen them both recently for minor ailments, on separate occasions. You discover that Richard has made an appointment today with the practice phlebotomist.

It is not unusual for a GP to be asked to take samples for patients on behalf of other bodies. This particular request is unusual for most GPs. From the information available, the GP can only guess at the reason, the most likely being to confirm or disprove paternity. The result could have significant consequences for the patient and his wife.

Bearing in mind the requirements for explicit consent, how ought this situation to be managed?

Protecting patients

Ethical principles of beneficence and justice

The closeness and constancy of the relationship between GPs and their patients offers the GPs the privilege of learning much about their backgrounds, their families, their hopes, disappointments and expectations. Rarely, the GP may become suspicious of some irregularity of which the patient is unaware. It is only a suspicion, but if true, it provides a threat to the patient's welfare in some way. An elderly patient acquiesces in living arrangements which may suit both the patient and her relatives – or the arrangements may be detrimental to her care whilst beneficial to them. Is there an ethical principle that entitles the GP to interfere?[17]

Mrs Thomas is 90 years old and is resident in a nursing home, where she appears content. Her mental and physical frailty means that her GP needs to see her most weeks whilst visiting the home. The GP has met Mrs Thomas' only living relative, a niece by marriage, once or twice, whose attitude to her aunt seemed uncaring; also she was quite aggressive towards the GP. The next time the GP visits the home, matron says that Mrs Thomas has been discharged home by her niece, against her advice. Matron has been told that a private nurse is to be employed to look after Mrs Thomas at home, and there is no need for the GP to call. She is very concerned about these arrangements, in view of Mrs Thomas' general condition.

It can be very difficult to know how to deal with suspicions, as yet unfounded. They may be grounded in a dislike or mistrust of someone else's attitude or motives. A true appraisal of the situation is likely to be affected by these negative impressions. It can be helpful to discuss concerns with others who may confirm such impressions.

In this case, the matron has concerns about her patient's future welfare that she has transmitted to the GP, who may have similar doubts. Unlike the matron, the GP has a continuing responsibility for Mrs Thomas' medical care, but is frustrated in providing this by the niece's probable refusal to admit the GP to the house.

Ought the GP to be curious about the niece's motives in making these arrangements? Mrs Thomas may be very well looked after in her own home by a resident trained nurse: there may be every intention on the niece's part to ask the GP to call if or when medical assessment and treatment becomes necessary. If this is the case, the niece's motives are not relevant. It is in the GP's mind that the responsibility for proper supervision of the quality of care for Mrs Thomas lies with him, and as things stand, he has no way of fulfilling that responsibility. The fear might be that at some future time he could reproach himself by saying 'You knew it was going on but you did nothing to stop it.'

Special relationships

Other doctors

In an ideal situation, all the doctors who share the healthcare of a particular patient communicate with each other; all the relevant information is shared between them as well as with the patient. This is an area of communication of which most patients are fully aware, and with which they agree; it is after all to their benefit.

At times, the GP will become aware that the situation is less than ideal – letters go astray, telephone messages are not relayed, the patient is called upon to act as messenger, or go-between. It can prove difficult to decide which doctor is clinically responsible for which treatment – and meanwhile the patient trusts that everyone is making his or her own appropriate contribution to his care.

Valerie is a new patient whose previous records have not yet arrived in the practice. She tells her GP that she is about to start taking clomiphene that was prescribed for her by another doctor. It becomes clear that she does not remember being told by the prescribing doctor about potential side effects or precautions that she should take, in fact, she is certain she was told nothing. She has an appointment to see the other doctor in 3 months' time.

Valerie is currently unaware of her possible exposure to risk, however small the risk might be. It is immaterial whether she has already been given any information at all: the important thing is that even if she has, she has not retained it. It is likely that she trusts her doctor to ensure her safety and not to ask her to take any medication that might harm her. She may have subconsciously discounted any information that indicated that the treatment might be damaging rather than helping her towards a successful outcome. In any case, her new GP is poised to threaten her trust in another doctor – or to leave her ignorant.

How ought the GP to handle this situation?

Doctors and doctors' families as patients

We could say that objectivity is important when treating a patient. By this we mean the ability for the doctor to see beyond all the personal confounding elements in a consultation in order to empathise with the patient and produce a clear-sighted conclusion. There are some patients who, through no fault of their own, threaten this objectivity. In this group we might include close friends as well as other doctors and their families. It is for this reason that GPs are well advised not to treat their own families, nor their GP partners, nor even the practice staff. Yet all doctors as well as their families will need medical care from a colleague at some time. The question arises: how does the GP compensate for these obstacles to clear thinking?

There is a general awareness among GPs that everyone has on their list some patients who are popularly termed 'heart sink' for a variety of reasons – frequent attendance, unsatisfactory outcomes, lack of progress, indeed, any characteristic that induces a feeling of failure in their doctor (*see* Chapter 5). When such patients move away the sense of relief in the GP lasts only until each is replaced by a new one. A similar feeling of unease in the consultation may prevail between a GP and his medical patient, if for different reasons.

The ethical consideration for these interchanges must be the will to maintain patient autonomy without being overwhelmed by outside pressures or undermined by the patient's wish to be in total control.

Walter has recently retired as a GP. He has been self-medicating for his hypertension for many years through the dispensary at his own practice. This is no longer possible. He drops a note to his own GP whom he has not seen for some time, asking for a repeat prescription. His GP notes that his last recorded blood pressure was very high. Walter has so far ignored repeated requests to attend the surgery for review.

It is tempting to make the assumption that the more knowledgeable the patient, the less need there is for the GP to attempt either to impose control, to educate and inform, or merely to act as supervisor of the patient's medical care. The need for the GP to take over a more active role is evident when the patient appears to be making choices that are difficult for the GP to overlook. Is Walter's GP entitled to assume that Walter is well aware of the long-term effects of uncontrolled hypertension and can make a properly informed choice about his own blood pressure levels and appropriate medication? Yet he is being asked to condone this choice by continuing to prescribe for an otherwise non-compliant patient.

It could be that Walter is attempting to communicate with his own medical adviser, his GP, on the same level as previously he might have communicated with another medical colleague on behalf of a mutual patient. In order to 'save' his own GP time and trouble he regards himself as the 'mutual patient'. He may not realise that this misconception relies on unsafe practice by his GP and will threaten to undermine the GP's own professional integrity.

The public view

The continuing media publicity regarding 'bad doctors' is greeted with concern by the medical profession. A steady trickle of reporting about GPs who betray their patients' trust and behave in quite unacceptable ways is having the same effect. It is yet to become clear whether in fact the public's trust in their GPs is threatened seriously and irrevocably. There is a natural tendency for over-reaction on the part of the medical profession and politicians, yet the GP's responsibility to the community does not change, nor do his duties to patients.

Paternalism power and conflict: 'hard cases'

Ethical principles of respecting autonomy and justice

Every day the GP will face specific problems with particular groups of patients that will pose seemingly unanswerable ethical questions.

The very sick

When someone succumbs to a serious illness, however briefly, that person's autonomy is often diminished for a time. Reasoning and competence to make decisions may be well maintained, yet the patient expresses a desire to delegate decisions on treatment to the 'expert' – the GP.

Can this be regarded as a fully autonomous decision? Or is the GP being coerced into an ethically inappropriate paternalistic role by the patient?

Over-dependency

There are some people, the most obvious examples being those with psychologically based physical symptoms, who derive great benefit from counselling in the practice. Many GPs are able to help patients to resolve their problems in this way. This activity can prove very satisfying for the GP, particularly if there is a good response.

Yet at what stage does a steady increase in dependency on the GP begin to erode a patient's self-reliance and autonomy?

Value judgements (*see* Chapter 10)

People who smoke, people who are obese, anyone whose choice of lifestyle does not conform to the accepted view of 'healthy', runs the risk of being discriminated against. They will have a shorter life span than the rest of the population: but it is because they are more likely to suffer debilitating and disabling disease that they are also more likely to be frequent visitors to the GP surgery. At the same time, GPs have been allotted the task of influencing them and making them change their habit, a task that tends to be a poorly rewarded activity in terms of success. The smoker is probably fully aware on the one hand that his recurrent chest problems are related to his smoking, but on the other he says he 'cannot' give up smoking. He still smokes, and he still comes to see the GP to get the prescription he needs for bronchitis or obstructive airways disease. Many similar examples could be quoted – smokers with peripheral vascular disease or angina, the overweight with arthritic knees or poorly controlled diabetes.

Discrimination against this group of patients is most likely to occur in the debate on rationing of scarce resources which has now extended into general practice. Utilitarian distribution would demand that resources go first to those who would benefit most, and thereby produce most value for money spent. This is the theory underlying the proposal that each intervention be measured in terms of Quality Adjusted Life Years, or 'QALYs' (*see* Chapter 10). It is difficult to maintain an argument which supports the plea that someone was refused treatment *solely* because he was a smoker, or too fat: there is little distinction that can be made between a treatment decision made on clinical grounds and one made on grounds of lifestyle – the two are too closely connected. The outcome of knee surgery in an obese person is better if weight is lost prior to surgery and similarly, the benefit to a smoker of coronary artery surgery will last longer if he gives up smoking. Decisions to make access to surgical treatment conditional on a change in lifestyle are common and are said to be made on clinical grounds. They could also be viewed as discriminating against these patients and therefore unjust. We might include the question of access to drug treatment. The introduction of new drugs that are claimed to help the obese to lose weight and smokers to stop smoking has given rise to further controversy.

Ought justice to prevail, and allow all patients equal access to surgery, and prescription of these drugs to smokers and the obese, albeit at a certain cost to the health service, arguing that the benefit to this section of the population outweighs the cost? Or ought it to be the utilitarian principle that governs the distribution of these resources by targeting preferentially those whose lifestyle does not compromise the treatment outcome?

Patients' beliefs

Some people have beliefs about health and disease that are eccentric or unusual. Others have a religious or ethnic culture that differs markedly from that in Britain. The GP may find himself in difficulties if he is ignorant of this; these patients will not necessarily accept or comply with current accepted medical practice.

Mr Young is 74 years old and troubled by a disabling tremor. The consultant neurologist has diagnosed Parkinson's disease and has started him on appropriate medication. He comes to see his GP complaining that he is no better. On further questioning he says he does not believe in taking the tablets and has thrown them away. He has been to a clairvoyant who has told

> him that he ought to seek help from the spirits rather than from
> tablets. He makes it clear to the GP that he believes what the
> clairvoyant has told him.

Many patients consult practitioners of alternative medicine, some
to good effect. The interface between alternative and traditional
medicine is unclear, particularly when patients with serious conditions relinquish traditional evidence-based treatment for less well-
researched alternatives. On occasion, a patient's decision appears so
irrational as to cast doubt on his mental stability. Mr Young's adviser
could not be categorised as an alternative therapist, but nevertheless, has had a substantial influence on the patient's attitude to conventional medicine.

In similar situations, does the GP honour the patient's autonomous decision or attempt to override it? (*See* Chapters 5 and 6.)

The elderly

Similar questions arise with treatment of the elderly, although advancing age is beyond anyone's control, unlike a lifestyle choice. The
ethical principle of justice, which aims for equality for all, might be
awkward to sustain where it becomes necessary to make hard distributive choices between the young and the old. For example, is it
reasonable to restrict referrals for coronary artery surgery to those
under a certain age? If there are no age restrictions, the older patient
could be taking the place of a younger person who has years of
useful work in front of him and a young family to support.

The theoretical ethical dilemma runs thus:

- on the one hand, the young person has many years to live. The
  treatment will restore him to good health in order to contribute
  positively to the good of society. In general, treatment has more
  chance of success in the younger age group where the basic phy-
  siological systems function well. Therefore the resource decision
  ought to favour the young
- conversely, although the expectation of life for the old person
  may be short, enhancing the quality of that life, however short,

is important in maintaining independence in old age. An independent person is very much less a burden to society compared to a dependent person. An old person has already made a substantial contribution to the good of society during his life. He has earned the right now to claim his deserts in the form of medical treatment.

It is uncomfortable to contemplate such stark choices: ideally, it ought to be possible for each individual to be treated according to their needs, not preferentially according to their age or other personal characteristic. We know that health costs and demands on the GP rise with advancing age: this is reflected in the cash loading for the care of elderly patients on the GP's list. We should also take into consideration that this section of the population is less demanding and more accepting of shortcomings in healthcare; if complaints are made, they are most often made by concerned relatives or carers on the old person's behalf rather than by the patient himself.

The 1990 GP contract required GPs to invite all patients over 75 years old for an annual health check. This was probably a well-intentioned attempt to promote better health in this age group in spite of the fact that there was little evidence that such an exercise would be beneficial; many GPs regarded it as wasteful of time and resources. It does, however, raise an ethical question: does the GP have any greater duty to the elderly to protect their rights to intensive healthcare than to the younger patients on his list?

Caring for drug-dependent patients (*see* also Chapter 5)

Patients who are drug-dependent experience difficulty in being accepted onto a GP's list. This is for a variety of reasons: for example, the GP's lack of expertise in this area of medicine and the time needed to devote to the problems such patients bring to the surgery. There are other more nebulous reasons: the fear of disruption in the surgery, behaviour upsetting to other patients, non-compliance with advice or medication, anticipated violence and criminal behaviour, lack of continuity of care due to shifting addresses, and a host of others.

This is a group of people within society whose rights to the continuity of healthcare provided in general practice are equal to those of the rest of the population. As Dicker points out, primary care is the most accessible source of help for substance abusers, and refusal to treat them in primary care is a failure of the minimum duty of doctors:

> At best the failure to offer treatment for drug users in practice is unethical. At worst it represents a dereliction of the moral duty of doctors to their potential patients and a failure to grasp a unique opportunity to confer a benefit to the society of which they are a part.[18]

This is a strong statement: its veracity will depend on the recognition of its roots in deontology – the duty of a doctor, and the utilitarian view of benefit to society as a whole.

This representation is endorsed by the GMC with the unequivocal statement that treatment of opiate addiction in general practice is part of the job. Thus:

> you must not allow your views about a patient's lifestyle, culture, beliefs, race, colour, gender, sexuality, age, social status, or perceived economic worth to prejudice the treatment you provide or arrange.[19]

Yet it is *because* of their habit, that of dependency on drugs, that many are in effect 'outlawed'. Drug dependency may bring with it poverty, aggression and criminality, but it is also associated with well-recognised substantial health problems and incidence of disease. It could also affect a person's autonomy by overwhelming free will and self-determination – the desire for drugs becoming the most important aspect of life.

Can the present reluctance on the part of many GPs to accept substance abusers on to their lists be morally justified?

Conclusion

We have seen that a GP's professional duties to his patients are of fundamental importance. The GP has a duty to provide an acceptable standard of care for his patients; an understanding of the ethical components of the interaction between patient and GP is crucial to the quality of care that the patient receives.

References and notes

1   Extract from Carver R (1990) What the doctor said. In: *A New Path to the Waterfall*. Collins Harvill, London, p. 149.

2   Mill JS (1962) On liberty. In: M Warnock (ed.) *Utilitarianism*. Harper Collins, Glasgow, p. 188.

3   This is planned according to the revalidation consultation document circulated by the General Medical Council in May 2000.

4   *Collins English Dictionary* (1994) HarperCollins, Glasgow.

5   Dr Harold Shipman, convicted of murdering patients.

6   General Medical Council (1998) *Maintaining Good Medical Practice*. GMC, London, p. 6.

7   Montgomery J (1997) Professional regulation. In: *Health Care Law*. Oxford University Press, Oxford.

8   There are new powers assigned to the GMC under amendments to the Medical Act 1983 that came into force on 3 August 2000. These have been designed to address some of the criticisms of the workings of the GMC's professional conduct committee.

9   This is set out in the series of booklets produced by the GMC since 1995 under the general title *Duties of a Doctor*. Individual booklets are referred to throughout this book.

10 The anaesthetist who voiced his concerns about the outcome of paediatric cardiac surgery at Bristol was subsequently unable to get a job in the UK.

11 The secretary of the local medical committee is the usual contact point for a GP.

12 General Medical Council (1998) *Good Medical Practice*. GMC, London, paras 23–4.

13 This does not mean to say that this should *never* happen. Many procedures have been carried out in wartime without the benefit of properly conducted trials – for example, the use of penicillin.

14 This is recognised in the motto of the Royal College of General Practitioners, 'Cum Scientia Caritas', translated as 'scientific knowledge applied with compassion'.

15 Leydon GM, Boulton M, Moynihan C *et al.* (2000) Cancer patients' information needs and information seeking behaviour: in depth interview study. *BMJ*. **319**: 909.

16 A policy of paying doctors for their time spent in explaining the nature of a patient's medical condition and treatment plan has been brought in by the Japanese Ministry of Health and Welfare. Akabayashi A and Fetters MD (2000) Paying for informed consent. *J Med Ethics*. **26**: 212–14.

17 In Guy de Maupassant's *The Devil* he tells the story of Honore the farmer and his 92-year-old mother who is very ill. The doctor is called and insists

that Honore must not let his mother be left alone. But the good July weather demands that Honore gets out in the fields and harvests his wheat. He employs the local terminal care nurse on a fixed price contract to look after his mother until she dies. The nurse works out that if the old woman dies soon she will make a profit. She frightens the old woman to death by dressing up as the devil. The nurse makes her profit and the son gets his crops planted. *Boule de Suif and other stories* translated by Sloman HNP (1940) Penguin, Harmondsworth.

18 Dicker A (1999) Obligations of general practitioners to substance mis-users. *J R Soc Med.* **92**: 422–4.

19 GMC (1998) *Good Medical Practice.* General Medical Council, London. para. 13.

CHAPTER THREE

Confidentiality: 'Your secret is safe with me'

Summary

The duty of confidence is inherent in every patient–doctor contact. This duty is based on important ethical principles and is considered under the following headings, together with the relevant legal background:

- In the consulting room
- Patient records
- The practice team
- Outside agencies
- Protection of others
- GP education.

Whatever, in connection with my professional practice, or not in connection with it, I see or hear, in the life of men, which ought not to be spoken of abroad, I will not divulge, as reckoning that all such should be kept secret. (See Appendix 1.)

Personal information consists of those facts, communications, or opinions which relate to the individual and which it would be reasonable to expect him to regard as intimate or sensitive and therefore want to withhold or at least to restrict in their collection, use or circulation.[1]

Introduction

Ethical principles: non-maleficence, autonomy, justice

The first ethical principle that relates to the duty of confidence is that of *non-maleficence*. The GP is in a privileged position: there is much that he knows about each patient that has been given to him in confidence. The patient will feel betrayed if the GP he trusted did not keep his confidence secure.[2] Actual damage – to a relationship, to employment, or to social status – could occur, but less obvious harm, or potential harm, could be equally concerning to the individual.

Secondly, it is important to understand the exceptions to the rule of confidence, particularly where the patient benefits. The *autonomous* patient will be able to consent to information being given to others, and may be quite specific as to what may be passed on, and what is to remain confidential. It would be morally wrong to ignore the right of a patient to give or withhold such consent.

Thirdly, societal *justice* demands that where serious harm may be prevented by disclosure without consent, the doctor has an obligation to disclose.

The relationship between patient and doctor is based on trust. The patient relies on the doctor to protect him from harm, as well as to provide help in his distress. Any breach of the patient's confidence may lead to harm, and sometimes patients are very fearful of this. If the doctor can reassure his patient that all information regarding that patient remains confidential, then the patient will feel at ease when giving very sensitive, and sometimes troubling, details to the doctor. The inherent quality of such private information places the doctor under an obligation *not to divulge* it. In line with Hippocrates, the doctor must not breach confidence without the patient's consent.

The *deontological* view, that proposed by Immanuel Kant, upholds the sense of duty to others when preserving the privacy of information. It is a rule that is rational as well as intuitive, and is of practical benefit to the individual. It is also important to be aware that patients rely on the medical culture that 'doctors don't tell'.

There are exceptions to this fundamental rule. The most obvious is the sharing of clinical information between different doctors involved in a patient's care. There are other exceptions which will be discussed later in this chapter. This is a necessity, and facilitates good clinical practice. It could be said that the patient's consent is implicit, particularly when a referral to another doctor is discussed in the consultation. It would also be implicit that the transmitted information is *relevant* to the referral. However, there are other situations where confidence is breached, either by accident, inadvertently, or intentionally but without the patient's consent. It is these situations which are potentially damaging, and involve actions which could be both ethically and legally reprehensible.[3]

In the consulting room

Privacy

Consultations in general practice are normally conducted in private, in a room with the door closed. Others, apart from the patient and the doctor, may be present, but this will only be with the consent of the patient. Sometimes a patient will ask the doctor for permission for another – spouse, friend, relative – to be present, clearly unaware that it is the patient's own consent that is required. On the other hand, the doctor will need to ask the patient for consent for a medical student or other medical observer in training to be present.[4]

Mr Allen, the headmaster of a nearby school, has approached your practice. Some sixth-form students are thinking of medicine as a career, and would like to spend a few days with local practices as observers. Ideally, he says, this would include sitting in on consultations. He assures the GPs that these are mature pupils who are fully aware of the need to preserve confidentiality.

The headmaster has the interests of his pupils at heart. He knows that if a student is well informed before deciding on a career, he or she will be more likely to make a reasoned choice. Medicine requires a more specific preparation at school than some other professions. He sees this experience as an opportunity to inform intending medical students in a practical way.[5]

His viewpoint could be recognised as valid. Career choices can be difficult to make, and the more a student knows about the practical aspects of medicine, for example, the more committed he will be. It would be a waste of resources if even a small number of undergraduate students fail to complete a course because it turned out to be very different from their expectations. Requests for work observation by prospective medical students in the sixth form are becoming more common, and the benefit must be weighed against the possible threat to patient autonomy, particularly where confidentiality may be compromised. Patients whose consultations were to be observed would have to give their consent for the pupil to be present. Any refusal would have to be honoured, and ought not to affect the content or outcome of the consultation.

On the other hand, an unforeseen request for such an exercise might have a profound effect on the unprepared patient's view of the impending consultation. At the very least, in agreeing, the patient's 'hidden agenda' is more likely to remain hidden. At most, the patient may refuse consent, but yet feel that he is impeding medical progress by doing so.

> How would you respond to Mr Allen, and what are the ethical arguments that influence your decision?

The content of the consultation

If a consultation is to have a beneficial outcome, the doctor needs to understand what it is that is troubling the patient. Therefore the patient needs to give the *whole* story. Even an outwardly straightforward physical symptom may have another important dimension, which may only be discovered by the doctor if the patient allows. The patient will withhold certain information if he feels that the doctor will tell others, or that it will be recorded in a place that is open to other eyes. The paper record, tucked away in its Lloyd

George envelope, has an air of privacy about it. Now that many practices are computerised, patients can see their records displayed on screen, and can watch as their GP enters information about them on that screen.

We could postulate that this development has encouraged a better balance of power in the consultation. GP and patient can agree on the content of the consultation, and the words best used to describe it. The GP and his computer are helping the patient to be more *autonomous*. We do not know, however, whether this method of record keeping, and the perceived loss of privacy, have inhibited the patient. What will the GP put on the record after the patient has left the room? More importantly, who else will see it?

Mrs Adams has come for a blood pressure check and a repeat prescription. Whilst the printer on the GP's desk is producing this for her, she asks for a repeat prescription for an inhaler for her 15-year-old asthmatic daughter, Alice. Alice's inhaler has run out and she needs another today.

If we assume that this GP is fully computerised, it will be very simple for him to bring up Alice's notes on the screen on his desk, and issue the repeat prescription to give to her mother. But maybe Alice is sexually active, and 'Gillick competent' (*see* Chapter 8); one of the doctors in the practice has recently started her on an oral contraceptive. She has the right to confidentiality. Although the GP will have encouraged her to involve her parents, she may not have done so yet. At this point, there is a risk that when Alice's records are displayed on the screen in front of her mother, her confidence will be compromised.

Sometimes when a couple registers with a GP the two individuals come for their new patient checks at the same time. In the consulting room each is privy to the other's responses to questions. Each may maintain that they 'have no secrets' to keep from the other. This is not invariably so, and the doctor will need to be sensitive to this. For example, a husband may be ignorant of his wife's history of a teenage termination of pregnancy; there could be sound clinical reasons why it would be helpful for the doctor to know of this, although the wife wishes it to be kept from her husband. The doctor must be aware that the whole medical history can take time to emerge.

Third party encounters

Patients' relatives and friends sometimes come to see the GP, either with information to impart, or with requests for information from the doctor. Often the patient is unaware of this contact, and just as often, the third party will say that they are only doing this, or asking for that, because they have the patient's 'best interests' at heart. (*See* Chapter 6 for the incompetent adult patient and Chapter 8 for children.)

> Betty comes to see the GP complaining of a sore throat. The GP takes a swab. She says she will phone for the result. She asks the GP not to contact her at her home. She has left her husband, Bernard, for good, and is staying with friends. She tells the GP that he has been physically aggressive to her over a long period of time. She appears calm and rational. She refuses the GP's offer of referral to a counsellor. Bernard phones the next day. He says Betty has been behaving strangely for some time, and that she is asking for a referral to a psychiatrist. He says she has told him of her visit to the surgery yesterday, and she doesn't want to come up yet again. He asks the GP to arrange the referral.

The two stories, as told by Betty and Bernard, conflict with each other. On the basis of the information that Betty has given her GP, together with her demeanour, the GP might regard Betty as a rational, self-determining person, with a right to preservation of her confidence. Her reason for telling the GP of her marital situation is straightforward and practical: she is protecting the GP from at best, a wasted phone call, and at worst, an unpleasant rebuff from Bernard. But Bernard sounds genuinely concerned, and anxious to do the best for his wife. The GP is constrained from detailed questioning of Bernard, being conscious of the necessity to protect Betty's confidence. Yet he now wonders if he gave Betty enough time yesterday, to expand on her story.

> What might be your response to Bernard, outlining the ethical reasoning governing that response?

Patient records

The verbal interchange between patient and doctor, if conducted in the privacy of the consulting room, can remain confidential, if both agree. There is much that is transferred from patient to doctor which is never recorded formally, but which contributes to the development of the ongoing relationship and understanding. But once information is recorded on paper or electronically, it is possible that others can have access to it.

Who owns the record?

Is it the doctor, on whose premises the record is stored, or who owns the electronic equipment? Is it the health authority, who has provided the paper used for the record? Or is it the patient, who provides the basis of the information in the record? It could be said that *ownership* of the record is unimportant.[6] It is the *use* of the information in the patient record that is of importance, both ethically and legally. The record-holder is under an obligation of confidence which overrides any question of ownership. It is the preservation of the patient's confidentiality that is paramount. Thus, even if the health authority claims to own the medical record, its contents could not be released to that authority without the patient's consent. We know that the full patient record is returned to the HA when that patient transfers to another GP. The HA becomes the record-holder, and is then bound by the rules of confidentiality.

The function of the medical record

We have seen how it is necessary for the patient to trust the doctor to preserve his confidence in the consultation. He also needs to trust the GP to keep accurate records of his medical history. This is in order that now and in the future the details of symptoms, investigations, diagnoses, and management are accessible to whoever needs to know. How much detail to record will depend on the condition described. It is important to bear in mind when entering material on the paper or computer record that the law supports the right of patients to view their medical records.[7] Few would welcome pejorative comments however true they might be.[8]

The patient will understand the main reason for keeping accurate medical records, which is to act as an aid to diagnosis and clinical management. It is obvious that results of clinical examination and laboratory tests must be recorded – no one would expect to rely on the memory of the GP. What may be less clear is the reason for recording more sensitive information and patients' personal confidences. The patient may ask that some information is withheld from the record, or even erased. This person is probably more aware than most of the number of intermediaries who can view the record, and who have access to their secrets. For example, every time a patient is referred to a consultant, the referral letter, if not the complete record, passes through many hands before landing up on the consultant's desk.

Colin asks the GP to erase all record of his alcohol consumption from his medical record. He says that he has decided that this should not be part of his medical record. The GP notes that the record referring to this aspect of his lifestyle is unremarkable.

How would you deal with his request?

Although you may be curious about the reason for Colin's request, he may not be forthcoming on this point. He seems to be asking you to respect his autonomy, and wishes to choose the content of his medical records. At some previous visit, he has clearly given the information to the recorder, whether nurse or GP, but has now changed his mind. The request may be unusual, but is there any good reason why you would not comply? And would you respond differently if the record indicated a high level of alcohol consumption? If Colin has the right to have an accurate entry erased, should not other patients have the same right?

The practice team

Exactly the same rule of confidentiality that binds the GP applies to each member of the practice team. The rule will have been introduced as part of the professional training of some members – in particular, the nurses and health visitors. It is the GP's responsibility, as employer, to ensure that all the other members of the team are aware of the importance of preserving patient confidentiality. It must form part of staff training, and there must be a specific confidentiality clause in the contract of employment. It is so important that a breach of patient confidence on the part of a member of staff could be a reason for summary dismissal.

Test results

The telephone is often a very useful method of communication. Patients will use it to make appointments, ask for advice or home visits, and get test results. Often they will transmit sensitive information about themselves to the person on the other end. The person may be a complete stranger – but nevertheless someone they look on as a trusted member of the practice team. It has become such an accepted way of communicating that its ethical pitfalls are forgotten.

> Debbie phoned the practice for the result of her pregnancy test. It was not immediately available, and a member of staff promised to find out the result and ring her back. By the time she did so, Debbie had gone out and left her answer phone on. The member of staff left the result of the test on the answer phone for Debbie to pick up on her return.

Patients need to know the results of tests. It would be impracticable for a busy practice always to insist that they attend the doctor or practice nurse for normal results, or that they are sent the results in the post. The telephone seems a useful tool in this area. But more and more people are relying on the answer phone to collect messages.

> Was the staff member guilty of a breach of confidence when she left the message on the answer phone in response to Debbie's request?

In the waiting room

The geographical layout of some practice buildings is not helpful in preserving patient confidentiality. An open-plan waiting room/ reception area gives an impression of friendliness and spaciousness at the same time. Patients can see the staff about their business, and the staff can keep an eye on the waiting room. Distressed or disabled patients can be supported, and explanations given to the waiting group when doctors run late. It does mean, however, that conversations can be overheard more easily, in particular, those at the reception desk or over the telephone. Inadvertent disclosure of confidential patient information can easily occur, and everyone in the practice needs to be aware of this.

HIV status

There are some areas of clinical practice that are particularly sensitive. The question will arise as to whether certain information ought to be kept confidential between doctor and patient. It may be that there are others in the practice who need to have access to this information, for the patient's benefit or for their own protection. The most obvious example of this is the HIV status of the patient. For example, does the practice nurse need to know this before she treats a patient?[9]

We could say that there are sensible precautions to avoid needle stick injuries that should be taken by all practitioners, doctors and nurses alike, for each and every patient. This is an example of good medical practice. On the other hand, we could also suggest that a practitioner is failing in his duty to his colleagues and members of staff if he withholds information about a patient that might put them at high risk of injury.

There is now a legal and moral obligation for doctors themselves to be open about their HIV status. This is in order to protect the patients in their care. Is there an equal obligation placed on the patient? There is a particular difficulty surrounding this clinical area and doctors and patients sometimes go to much greater lengths to preserve confidentiality for this than for many other areas of healthcare (*see* p. 55).

Colleagues and neighbours

Some practices will have members of staff or even partners registered in-house. Although this arrangement is generally considered to be inadvisable, nevertheless it still occurs. Indeed, in rural and sparsely populated areas it would be difficult to avoid. This raises the question of how the confidentiality of these particular patients is to be maintained. It may in fact be impossible to do so and everyone in the practice needs to be aware of this. This is an administrative issue rather than an ethical one, the ethics depending on the confidentiality rules having already been laid down.

> Elaine has come to discuss contraception with the GP. She has not needed this for some time; a few years ago the GP remembers referring her husband for his vasectomy that was then successfully performed. She asks the GP not to record anything about this consultation in her notes: one of the practice's receptionists is their near neighbour.

Elaine has a dilemma. She needs the GP's help, and is demonstrating her trust in the GP by coming to see him rather than going to the family planning clinic. However, although she may be able to trust her GP, clearly she has some reservations about the practice staff. The GP may be unhappy about the omission of this information from the patient record, merely from the good communication aspect. Others in the future may need to know the content of his clinical examination and management, for the patient's own benefit.

Elaine has made it very clear that the content of this consultation is especially confidential. Her GP has a duty of care towards her but may regard her request as indicative of her own disregard of the preservation of family relationships; his values may be very different from hers.

> What ethical arguments do you use in your response to Elaine's plea?

Use of patient data

It is not only the clinical content of the medical record that is subect to the rule of confidentiality. Basic patient data will be held in the practice that recalls not only names, dates of birth, National Health Service numbers, but also addresses and postcodes. If a particular group of patients is to be targeted for any reason, it is a simple matter to produce a list of that group of patients. We already have the example of the cervical screening system, where letters are sent from the health authority (HA) to women who become due for repeat smear tests.

Other data is also recorded in the patient file. Family history, smoking, drinking and exercise habit, all form part of this record.

> Frances, the health visitor, wants to set up some 'stop smoking' meetings for young girls. She is of the opinion that preventive measures in this age group would be of benefit later on when this group are starting their families: they might be less likely to smoke during pregnancy. She asks if the practice will give her a list of all the 16–18-year-old female smokers in the practice, so that she can send them invitations.

This sounds as if it is an eminently commendable project. The smoking habit in girls sets in at a young age, and tends to be persistent. These girls tend not to be frequent visitors to the surgery – at least, not until they want to go on the contraceptive pill. Even then, knowing that the pill and smoking do not mix well in health terms, few give up the habit. By the time they are ready to start on their first wanted pregnancy, smoking is part of their life.

Frances is an enthusiastic and dedicated professional. She sees the effects of smoking in families and on young children. Here is an ideal opportunity for her to use her expertise for their benefit, and to make some impact on the health of the community. No one, let alone a professional colleague, would wish to stand in her way. Indeed, is there any good reason why she should not have the list?

Yet the data collected about each patient is confidential, and this includes *all* the data. The ethical question is whether the data to be released to another health professional is with the patient's consent and for the patient's own benefit.

> The practice refuses Frances' request. What might be the ethical justification for this decision? Do you disagree, and if so, why?

Outside agencies

The GP receives a steady flow of requests from outside agencies for the release of information from the patient record held by the GP. Most often these requests are ostensibly for the benefit of the patient, but occasionally may be in conflict with the interests of that patient.

Requests can come from the:

- insurance companies – for preliminary medical reports (PMRs)
- solicitors
- medical researchers
- medical data handlers
- Benefits Agency (EB113)
- Driving Licensing Authority (DVLA)
- HA (for post-payment verification)
- visiting team for GP vocational training accreditation.

And probably in the near future from the:

- clinical governance evaluation team
- reaccreditation team.

The material requested is various, as is the indication of the individual patient's consent to the release of this material. Some written requests, for example, those from insurance companies, will include a copy of the patient's consent on a standard form, others give no indication of this. A fee will be paid to the GP for some responses and not for others.

When asked to provide information about patients to others there are three key principles to be followed. These form the ethical and legal basis for the protection of patients' confidentiality and are stated by the General Medical Council.

- Seek patients' consent to disclosure of information wherever possible, whether or not you judge that patients can be identified from the disclosure.
- Anonymise data where unidentifiable data will serve the purpose.
- Keep disclosures to the minimum necessary.[10]

In the case of post-payment verification, the HA visiting team, which may include non-medical personnel, will ask to see a random sample of patient records. If all the patients on the GP's list have been informed of this possibility and have full understanding that their medical records may be used in this way, then it is simple to identify those that have refused consent. Their records would be withheld from this exercise. If this is not the case, it is important that patient consent is obtained prior to scrutiny by the visiting team.[11]

There are three ethical issues here:

1 Patient consent (*see* also Chapters 2 and 6): is it explicit and informed, is it implicit, or is it undeclared?
2 Release of confidential information: is it for the patient's benefit?
3 Payment of fees: for whom is the GP acting, patient or fee-payer?

Specific examples

Lifestyle questions in PMRs

Requests for reports from the GP by insurance companies come to the GP at frequent intervals. They need to be dealt with reasonably quickly: undue delay may jeopardise the provision of an important insurance policy for the patient. The proposer's signed consent to release of information comes with the set of forms – but does the signatory know exactly what information his GP is being asked to provide?[12] Most companies ask for smoking and alcohol history, family history – sometimes listing specific genetic disorders[13] – but also human immunodeficiency virus (HIV) status, attendance at STD (sexually transmitted disease) clinics, and so on.

Where does the GP's responsibility lie? He is collecting a fee from the insurance company for completing the form, but he has a responsibility to his patient to protect his confidence. The validity of the patient's consent is in real doubt *unless* he knows in advance the questions the GP is to be asked to answer.

Geoff's girlfriend Gina comes to see the GP. She tells the GP that Geoff has been to the local STD clinic, and was told that she now needed to see her own GP for some 'tests' as they had found that he had an infection. Geoff himself has recently registered with the practice but has not been to the surgery yet, although his records have come through from his previous GP. Today's post has brought a request for a PMR for him, together with his signed consent form. The PMR includes the question 'Has the proposer ever attended a clinic for sexually transmitted diseases?'

The GP has no reason to doubt Gina's word. Also he knows that patients attending STD clinics are asked their permission before the clinic can communicate with the GP, and can refuse. There is, therefore, no reason for the GP to expect to hear from the clinic about Geoff's attendance.

How do you answer the question on Geoff's PMR form?

Requests from solicitors

It is becoming increasingly common for solicitors to ask the GP for *complete* sets of an individual's medical records, in order to settle litigation. Usually these come from the patient's solicitor, but occasionally they come from the opposing side. Often, when looking through the patient's records, the GP may be at a loss to understand the relevance to the case of some of the contents of the Lloyd George envelope, let alone the reel of paper which is the computer print-out. Medical records directly referring to the mishap, or accident, are the most clearly relevant, but how does the GP respond where the rest of the record contains bizarrely irrelevant material?

> Hannah suffered a back injury in a fall at work about 3 years ago. She has been unable to work since the accident, and has had an extensive rehabilitation programme that is ongoing. Her mental state has suffered; she is reacting badly to her disability and is clinically depressed as well. She is suing her employer, who is resisting the claim. The GP receives a request from her employer's solicitor, together with her signed consent, for *all* her medical records.

Many patients are unaware of the detailed content of their medical records. Hannah's record envelope may contain much that is trivial – episodes of minor illness, old laboratory reports, blood pressure recordings at times of contraceptive pill checks. There may also be recorded episodes that Hannah herself would consider much more confidential, but had forgotten about when she signed her consent for the solicitor.

> When the GP looks through Hannah's records, he finds that 10 years ago Hannah attempted suicide when a relationship broke up. There are several letters in her records from the psychiatrist whom she saw after this event. She was treated and followed up for 6 months, then discharged as fit.

> How ought you to deal with the solicitor's request?

Research projects

Research in general practice is an important way in which to develop an evidence base relevant to primary care. There have already been several valuable research projects that have utilised data collected from several large practices. There is usually a GP co-ordinator, who may ask for the GPs or staff within a practice to assist. More often, there will be someone from outside the practice who will need to access patient data for use in the project.

Sometimes, the outside researcher will wish to interview individual patients. In this case, the GP is able to identify specific patients and to obtain their explicit consent for the interview. The aim of the project can be explained and the patient's questions answered. The patient is given the opportunity to decline as well as to accept. Confidentiality is respected and the patient's autonomy preserved.

Other projects may require the collection of information from patient records. Epidemiological studies rely on the collation of large quantities of such data. The benefit of such studies to the general population, if conducted scientifically, can be very great. Yet has each patient given explicit permission for their personal confidential medical record to be used in such a way? And if asked, would a patient view a researcher from outside the practice differently from a GP, nurse or other member of the practice staff?

Dr Ingram is setting up a research project on back pain in the Region. He is interested in the information and advice that patients are given on the self-management of first episodes of uncomplicated back pain and their compliance with that advice. He writes to the practice asking for help with his research. His colleague, Irene, is a physiotherapist with an interest in back pain rehabilitation. She intends to visit all the practices included in the project and, using the practice database, search through the medical records to identify patients suitable for inclusion. She will then write to them asking for an interview.

Acute back pain is a common presenting symptom in general practice. Most episodes will resolve spontaneously in time, but can be very distressing for the patient and result in many days lost from work. This sounds as if it could be an interesting and useful project; if the research protocol that Dr Ingram has included with his letter appears sound, the practice might consider agreeing to the proposal. It is reassuring that neither the GPs nor the practice staff will be involved in any extra work. The GPs would probably wish to meet him and Irene to discuss the practical issues. However, there could be a problem with patient confidentiality. Ought consent to be obtained before Irene searches the records?

Reassurance on this point may have come with Dr Ingram's assurance that his project has been approved by the responsible research ethics committee. Guidance on this issue has been provided by the British Medical Association, with the proviso that:

> [w]here doctors are asked to release information for ethics committee approved research, but have doubts about whether the issues of confidentiality and consent to disclosure have been fully addressed, information should not be disclosed until the issue has been cleared up.[14]

A not altogether dissimilar problem arises when a GP is asked by an outside body to provide an update on a patient's condition.

> Jenny had a mastectomy for breast cancer at hospital X nearly 20 years ago. The GP gets a letter from Ms Jones in the breast unit at hospital X asking for a report on Jenny's current condition. The GP telephones Ms Jones and discovers that she describes herself as a 'data handler', and is updating the records in the unit.

The easiest response to both Dr Ingram and Ms Jones is to agree to the first and provide the report to the second. The intention of each is admirable. No one would wish to obstruct research or proper record keeping to the detriment of patient care. Yet each ignores the ethical necessity to protect the patient's confidentiality; a balance needs to be struck.

However, the GP's practice is in a position to be able to accommodate both requests – by identifying the study group for Dr Ingram among his patients, and contacting them personally, with full information on the project. In this way, each person is able to consent or refuse to take part, and the project can proceed.

Likewise, the GP is able to contact Jenny to ask for her permission to give Ms Jones the information she asks for, provided that Jenny will not be upset by such a request.

The use of anonymised patient data has recently been tested in the courts.[15] A company wished to obtain information on GPs' prescribing habits for commercial reasons. This would be done by downloading dispensing data from pharmacists' computers. Details about individual patients would already have been removed before the download, and the anonymised data would then be aggregated.

The company appealed against the initial judgement by Latham J, who had concluded that the proposed collection of such data would be 'a clear breach of confidence, unless the patient gives consent'.[16] The Latham judgement was viewed with much concern by all those involved in research and audit studies that relied on the use of aggregated anonymised patient information, for example, epidemiological studies. It went against the advice already published by the BMA.[17] 'The BMA believes that from an ethical perspective, disclosure or breach of confidentiality occurs only when the information revealed can be linked to a specific individual.' Fortunately, Lord Justice Simon Brown in the Court of Appeal allowed the company's appeal, saying that the 'concern of the law here is to protect the confider's personal privacy . . . [T]hat gives the patient no property in the information and no right to control its use provided only and always that his privacy is not put at risk.'

This is a clear instance where ethics and law are in agreement. Patient autonomy remains protected providing any data cannot be traced back to the individual, and no harm is done to that individual as a result – non-maleficence. The good which comes from properly conducted research using such data is not now threatened.

Protection of others

We have already established that patients trust their doctors to protect their confidence, and that the doctor–patient relationship relies on this to a large extent. This obligation of confidence laid on the doctor is upheld in law, but it is recognised that it is not an *absolute* obligation.[18] There is a special group of circumstances where there is a potential conflict between the protection of the patient's rights to confidentiality and the good of others.[19] The GP faces a difficult dilemma – whether to disclose, or not to disclose. He must decide in each individual case, weighing the likely benefit and harm in the balance. It is important to remember that another opinion, from a colleague or other medical agency, can be sought if the problem seems insurmountable.

Specific problems

Fitness to drive[20]

The first epileptic attack is significant, not only medically but also socially. If the patient is declared unfit to drive, this can have very unpleasant repercussions for him in his daily life. If the story is highly suggestive but not absolutely conclusive, the GP may feel pressured to adopt a 'wait and see' approach, at least until the neurologist has completed a full assessment. This could take many weeks and meanwhile the patient is still driving his car.

Alternatively, the GP may insist that the patient stops driving at once, at least until epilepsy has been ruled out. The recommendation by the GP for the patient to inform the Driver and Vehicle Licensing Authority (DVLA) and his insurance company is clear. There is, however, no confirmation that the patient has carried out the GP's instructions. Indeed, the GP may see the patient out in his car some time after the consultation.

The GP is in an invidious position. He has an indisputable responsibility to his patient to protect his confidentiality. Yet here is a situation which is potentially dangerous to other members of the public.

Keith is a sales rep. He comes to see the GP for a sick note. He tells the GP that he was taken to casualty a few nights ago with a cut head, having been knocked out at a party. The GP has already had a letter from the casualty officer who gives a slightly different story. He states that Keith was brought into casualty after an alcohol-induced fit.

This man depends on his car for his work. If he is banned from driving he will lose his job. He could well argue that he does not drink and drive, and if he only has a fit when he has been drinking, he is entitled to go on driving. If the GP is not persuaded by this argument, and insists that the DVLA must be told, Keith risks unemployment, with all its consequences for his wife and young family.

You advise Keith to stop driving, at least until he has had further investigations. You also ask him to inform the DVLA.

> He refuses, unconvinced by your arguments about his own safety and that of others. What do you feel you ought to do, if anything?

It may be helpful to consider how far the GP might be held responsible if Keith has a fatal accident whilst driving his car.

Transmissible disease

The example of the HIV positive man and his pregnant wife is now a well-known and often presented ethical dilemma. The GP knows of the positive result but the wife does not – and the husband refuses to tell her. Most people would now accept that the danger of her ignorance is too great to preserve his confidentiality, now that treatment and protection of the unborn child is a possibility. Should she be told, and is the benefit likely to outweigh the potential threat to family cohesion?[21]

Once again, this dilemma can only be resolved after the relative risks have been assessed. In this case, it is highly likely that the wife has been exposed to the risk of infection, and the child will also be at risk. Any suggestion that she could be tested specifically for HIV infection without her knowledge would clearly be morally unsound. Her informed consent would be necessary for such a procedure.[22]

It is important to be aware that as knowledge about the transmission and treatment of serious communicable disease advances, so does the moral argument become stronger in favour of disclosing information to those placed at serious risk. The protection of those at risk will override the responsibility to protect patient confidence.

Fertility treatment (*see* also Chapter 7)

The Human Fertilisation and Embryology Authority (HFEA) governs assisted fertility programmes in this country. It has produced a Code of Practice that includes consideration of the welfare of the child born as a result of fertility treatment.[23]

This requires treatment centres to 'satisfy themselves that the GP of each prospective parent knows of no reason why either of them might not be suitable for the treatment to be offered'. They are advised to obtain the parents' consent to approach the GP, and acceptance for treatment will depend both on this consent and on the GP's response. A 'clean' certificate would not be challenged, but some problem answers on the GP's form might jeopardise a couple's acceptance by the centre.

> Lawrence has two children from a previous marriage. Now divorced, he and his new wife Linda are seeking IVF after some years of infertility. Lawrence used to have an alcohol problem: once he threw his first child downstairs while he was drunk. The family problems at that time are clearly documented in his records. He says he has been teetotal ever since.

Is Lawrence's history relevant to his present situation? He and Linda may be desperate for help, and will do anything they possibly can to have a baby of their own. Linda may not even be aware of Lawrence's previous problem.

> Lawrence and Linda come to see you with their GP forms from the treatment centre, expecting you to complete them on the spot. Their long-awaited appointment for the centre is tomorrow. How do you respond to them?

This couple has already agreed to the centre approaching you, the GP, for information. They hope to realise their right to 'found a family' with your help. All you need to do now is complete the two forms, according to the records and the answers to questions you may need to ask.

Yet there are several important ethical problems hidden in this seemingly simple request.

1   Confidentiality – individual (Lawrence's history. Does Linda know?).
2   Confidentiality – as a couple. Does the treatment centre have a moral right to sensitive information as a condition of treatment? We do not apply these rules when giving preconceptual advice to our patients.

3   Duty of the GP to his patients, to protect them an ensure good treatment.
4   Duty of the GP to the future child.
5   Duty of the IVF centre to the future child.
6   Social justice – to administer funds for treatments in the way that society would endorse.
7   Professional responsibility of the GP not to withhold significant information.
8   Professional responsibility of the GP and of the centre *not* to make value judgements.

GP education

One of the most beneficial experiences of the GP registrar is that obtained through working with patients in the training practice. Observing others consult, then seeing and treating a wide variety of patients, together with discussion and review with the trainer, is a vital part of the vocational training programme.

The question of patient confidentiality arises in many aspects of GP education:

● case study discussion in day release courses
● use of video in training/assessment
● use of audio tapes in research projects
● research and audit projects
● publishing.

Case study discussion in day release courses

There is a long tradition in medical education of basing teaching on the clinical stories provided by real patients.[24] History, examination, investigations, treatment and outcome – there is something to be learnt from each and every 'case'.

Quoting once more from the BMA's document on confidentiality, '[t]eaching is an essential process but, in the BMA's view, it is contrary to the public interest to use identifiable material for teaching purposes without the subject's consent'.[25] The value of case discussion in the group is unquestioned: specific patients and their problems can provide a wide variety of learning matter for the GP registrars. The ethical question here lies with the words '*identifiable material*'. The patient's real name may be replaced by a pseudonym but age, sex and other social circumstances may all be crucial to the veracity of the story. It remains in doubt whether every patient is adequately anonymised before being presented to the group; there is also doubt that any have been asked to give their consent.

Is there then a moral argument for insistence on the observance of the BMA's recommendations *to the letter*? And what effect might this have on the learning experience of GP registrars?

Use of video in training/assessment

The acquisition of good consultation skills is considered vital to the teaching programme of the GP registrar. The consultation video is now being used as a valuable formative tool. The initial discomfort of seeing oneself on film seems to be overcome by most, and is recognised as worth overcoming for the benefit of learning. It is also used as part of summative assessment for the GP registrar, and is a component of the examination for membership of the Royal College of General Practitioners.

Although it is the GP who is learning from the video, or whose performance is being assessed by others, the patient is a clearly identifiable participant. This is one area of medical education where the utmost care is taken to obtain consent from the patient, both before the consultation and afterwards. There is the assurance that the film will only be used for teaching or assessment of the doctor, will be kept in a locked cupboard, and will be erased within one year. The patient is told that the recording is to be used 'to help teach doctors how to assess and improve their consultation skills and their ability to talk to patients.'[26]

The concern is no different from that produced by asking a patient to agree to the presence of an observer in the consultation. Is there an element of covert coercion, or is the consenting patient truly content to agree? Does the consenting patient then alter her agenda if the consultation is going to be less private than she had anticipated?

Use of audio tapes in research projects

The same ethical rules ought to apply. The sound of someone's voice may not seem to be quite so easily identifiable as their face on the screen – but the story they are telling is equally confidential, and that confidence needs to be respected. Those that have used audio tape in qualitative research have often found that the subject being interviewed will be surprisingly expansive in answers to questions. It is important to obtain consent as for the video tape, and that an assurance is given that the tape will be erased when the project is completed.

Publishing

However unlikely it may seem, an opportunity may arise for writing an article or a paper for publication. It is important to understand how easily patient confidentiality may be breached. Much that is of interest to the reader may contain anecdotal material that may be difficult to anonymise. Any attempt to make the patient's story less individual may mean that the paper loses its impact. However hard the writer tries to obscure the identity of a most interesting case, occasionally the attempt has not gone far enough, and someone identifies the patient.[27]

It is also often the case that the most powerful stories are provided by patients who might have difficulty in accepting any disclosure by giving consent, even if their stories were only to appear in a medical journal with a small professional circulation.

Reputable medical journals are specific about their rules on the use of patient material,[28] and the *BMJ* has produced a draft patient's consent form for use by authors.

Conclusion

The protection of a patient's confidence by the doctor is a fundamental element in the investment of trust in the doctor by a patient and is endorsed in the statement of a right to determine for yourself whether personal data may be disclosed and used. It is important that the GP adheres to the ethical principles that reinforce this right and understands that sometimes there needs to be a balance between individual autonomy and justice for the community.

References and notes

1   Wacks R (1994) *Personal Information: privacy and the law*. Clarendon Press, Oxford.

2   The European Group on Ethics in Science and New Technologies has asserted that personal health data form part of the personality of the individual.

3   The National Confidentiality and Security Advisory Body is to be set up in the UK to set national standards on confidentiality and security of patient information. The body will be multiprofessional and will include lay members – patients and the public.

4   The presence of a nurse as chaperone is normally accepted implicitly.

5   British Medical Association (1999) *Work Observation Guidelines*. BMA, London.

6   The Statutes relevant to medical records apply to the information held in such records, even though the medical record is held in law to be the property of the health authority (*see* Access to Health Records Act 1990 and Data Protection Act 1998).

7   Data Protection Act 1998 Chapter 29 Part II 'Rights of data subjects and others' 7(1).

8   In the Data Protection Act 1998, which came into force on 1 March 2000, patients have a new right to see *all* their medical records, paper and computer-held. Previously, this right only extended back to records made since 1 November 1991.

9   General Medical Council (1997) *Confidentiality: informing other health care professionals. 'Serious Communicable Diseases'*. GMC, London.

10   General Medical Council (2000) *Confidentiality: protecting and providing information*. GMC, London, para. 1.

11   *Ibid*. paras 14, 15, 29, 30.

12   The British Medical Association is currently working with the Association of British Insurers on the question of valid consent to disclosure.

13   It is common for a GP to look after whole families, so he will know of any family history of such disorders. In revealing this to the proposer's insurance company, he is breaching the confidence of other family members.

14 British Medical Association (1999) *Confidentiality and Disclosure of Health Information.*

15 R v Department of Health ex parte Source Informatics (1999) Court of Appeal December.

16 R v Department of Health ex parte Source Informatics (1999) **4** *All ER*: 185.

17 British Medical Association (1999) *Confidentiality and Disclosure of Health Information.* BMA, London, para. 3.4.

18 This was recognised by the Court of Appeal in W v Egdell (1990) *All ER*: 835, 848. This concerned a report on a mental patient held in a secure hospital. Disclosure of the patient's mental condition was held to be in a stronger public interest than that of protecting his confidence.

19 The exceptions to the general principle of preserving confidentiality are described fully in *Confidentiality and Disclosure of Health Information* (October 1999) British Medical Association. They include disclosure required by statute, disclosure in the public interest, and disclosure without consent in the subject's vital interests.

20 General Medical Council (2000) *Confidentiality: protecting and providing information.* GMC, London, paras 36–7.

21 General Medical Council (1997) *Serious Communicable Diseases.* GMC, London, para. 22.

22 *Ibid.* para. 4.

23 HFEA (1995) *Code of Practice*, para. 3.24.

24 There are some very detailed case histories of patients described as part of the research project carried out by Michael Balint and a group of GPs in 1956. Balint M (1964) *The Doctor, his Patient and the Illness* (2e). The Pitman Press, Bath.

25 British Medical Association (1999) *Confidentiality and Disclosure of Health Information.* BMA, London, para. 7.6.

26 Guidelines on a code of practice for videotaping of consultations – summative assessment: *Patient's consent form and information sheet* – Joint Committee for Postgraduate Training in General Practice VTSAB 1/7/99.

27 Smith R (1998) Informed consent: edging forwards (and backwards). *BMJ.* **316**: 949–51.

28 International Committee of Medical Journal Editors (1995) Protection of patients' rights to privacy. *BMJ.* **311**: 1272.

CHAPTER FOUR

Screening in primary care: whose risk is it anyway?

Summary

Whether prevention is actually better than cure is a question that needs to be addressed from the ethical perspective, as well as the practical. Screening is used as a vehicle to try to answer it.

- Definitions of screening and similar procedures
- Clinical good screening
- Morally good screening
- Role of beneficence
- Role of autonomy
- Application of utilitarian principles to screening
- Genetic screening
- Risk – an introduction
- Application of rights theory
- Manipulating populations
- Harms.

For disease cherishes a great longing for health, and health is the righteousness of body. Therefore disease will never be content with the possession of one organ already overcome, but will in fact send its noxious juices into all remaining organs.[1]

Introduction

This chapter is concerned with the need, or otherwise, of GPs to involve themselves in care of populations rather than individuals. We have discussed already the roots of the doctor's duties to individuals and how these duties emerged many centuries ago in various forms.

Inevitably, a legal duty to populations exists on the part of GPs because of statutory contractual rules. The 'list' of a GP defines the coverage of his or her duties. Strictly, there is only a duty to those who are signed onto the list of registered patients. The extent of the duty includes, among other things, the duty to offer a newly registered patient a check-up to include the measurement of their height and weight.[2] Thus all such patients, as a group, have a legally enforceable right to the measurement of their height by a suitably qualified practitioner. However, full examination of the appropriate statutory rules reveals that what the patient is entitled to, and what the doctor is obliged to deliver, is an assessment of weight and height for the calculation of Body Mass Index (BMI), as well as the identification of other risk factors such as those for ischaemic heart disease (IHD). This is in what is seen to be the patient's best interests.

> Is it right that government health authorities, by reference to the rules under which GPs work, should enforce this sort of screening?

Answering this question, and other similar questions that arise from the exercise of screening procedures, requires stepping back in the argument to examine the nature of screening a little more closely, and defining a few terms.

The nature of screening: contrasts in procedure

We can best describe *screening* as the search for presymptomatic or unidentified disease in a given population by various means: tests or examinations or other procedures. GPs in the UK are involved in many different screening exercises, for example:

- cervical cytology
- mammography
- testicular examination
- breast examination
- blood pressure measurement
- blood testing in pregnancy
- neonatal hip examination.

These examples include the screening of large populations to a given schedule, or *mass screening*, exemplified by the mammography programme; and *opportunistic screening*, where a GP takes the opportunity to suggest a measurement of, for example, blood pressure (BP) when the patient consults for some other reason.

A distinction should be drawn with the process of *surveillance*, which describes more than the simple application of a test or procedure to a well person. Surveillance implies a more complex activity which may involve some screening procedures but also clinical decision making and even diagnosis, with the participation of the patient or their agent. This might be exemplified by the routine preschool assessment of children's growth and development.

A further distinction should be made between both these activities and *chronic disease management* (CDM). For this, people with established disease are monitored to minimise the effects of that disease upon their health: asthma, diabetes and IHD are commonly followed in this way. It requires little further analysis to see CDM as beneficent.

Duties

Traditionally, doctors have responded to patients' needs for help in resolving their perceived illness; a duty has arisen from this relationship. That duty has been between the two people involved. Screening well people is different because no initial perceived problem has begun the relationship. The doctor has initiated the relationship because of the desire to perform a test in the best interests of the individuals of a group. In some circumstances the doctor is implementing state policy to do just that, and acting, it could be said, in the interests of the state.

In this way we begin to define a responsibility to a group. Were, for example, a woman not a member of a group of women aged between 20 and 65 on a GP's list, there would be no contractual responsibility on the doctor's part to provide cervical cytology services. The GP must offer a smear test to these women as a condition of service, representing a legally defined duty. But, in addition, there may be a moral responsibility to perform such a test, notwithstanding NHS policy.[3]

Good screening: practical justifications

Having used the description 'good', let us make some initial assumptions about what makes good screening in a search for what is ethically 'good'. We might say that a good screening programme reduces the burden of illness or death on a given population, with minimal side effects. This is a deceptively simple analysis and needs further examination to accommodate moral justification.

The World Health Organization (WHO) has developed a series of criteria which define good screening. These criteria address mainly the technical aspects of a process.[4]

Box 4.1   WHO screening principles

- The health issue should be important
- Treatment should be agreed by professionals for the benefit of sufferers
- Diagnosis and treatment facilities are available
- The illness should have an early symptomatic stage
- A diagnostic test exists
- The test should be acceptable to the population
- The illness has a well-understood course
- A policy exists on whom to treat
- Costs are appropriately balanced against other medical costs
- The process is sustainable

If it is accepted that the effectiveness of a programme is at least part of its ethical justification, it can be difficult to establish this in many situations, even with epidemiological help. Consider the following two examples.

Childhood neuroblastoma

Neuroblastoma is a severe, but rare, childhood cancer that can kill in early life, thus depriving its sufferers of a large number of useful years of existence. It is now possible to screen for this devastating condition by testing the urine for adrenaline metabolites. A positive test aids early diagnosis, yet it is known that in a proportion of children testing positive there will be a spontaneous remission. We need to ask whether the serious nature of the condition justifies screening the whole population at risk, given that the *overall* benefit to this group will be small.[5]

Cervical cytology

In contrast, the UK NHS cervical cytology screening programme screens about 4 million women per year, a vast enterprise for all concerned, not least the patients. Much has been written of the positive and negative effects of all this, and yet the exact role of this service has yet to be clarified. Undoubtedly, the cervical cancer death rate has fallen, probably due to a national call and recall system as described, but some experts in the field question this.[6]

> Is it necessary to have clear evidence of efficacy before accepting a system such as this as ethically sound?

It could be said that investment in a sound screening programme is worthwhile, and that prevention of serious or chronic illness is cost-effective. At first sight, it is intuitively correct that not to suffer an illness is better than suffering it. Consider this next example:

Lipids

Recent years have seen varying degrees of enthusiasm for screening of cholesterol blood levels in premorbid populations. There is a clear relationship between the development of IHD and intake of dietary saturated fats.[7] With the aim of reducing IHD rates, there are two possible interventions that could be applied to a population:

- they could be screened for high cholesterol levels to identify those at higher risk. This group could then be offered appropriate advice and drug therapy
- they could be offered dietary advice about reducing saturated fat intake in the form of a mass education campaign.

Whilst the aim is the same, the means are very different and quantifying the results is complex. The comparison is between the results of focusing on a high-risk group (identified through screening) and those of a mass encouragement strategy. Each of these strategies demands moral justification, as will be seen.

Good ethical screening

The case of phenylketonuria

So far, good screening has been described in a technical sense; this suggests that at least part of the ethical justification for screening rests on reliable methods and processes. To take this analysis a little further let us examine the other aspects of why it might be a good thing. Is it self-evident that prevention is better than cure?

For example, the screening of neonates by GPs or other members of the primary healthcare team includes the collection of a heel prick blood sample for detection of phenylketonuria (PKU), an in-born error of metabolism. PKU is a treatable condition. If food containing phenylalanine is excluded from the diet for at least 10 years, the child will develop normally. If there is no dietary exclusion PKU will lead to physical handicap and learning difficulties. Failure to screen is a cause of action in law: a recent case where a midwife did not screen for PKU led to a £2.5m out of court settlement.[8] It has an incidence of 1 in 16 000 (varying from 1 in 4000 in Scotland to 1 in 40 000 in Mexico).

What is the ethical background here?

Applying four ethical principles to PKU

We can see that the screening of a population for a preventable handicapping disease such as this using simple cheap identification is self-evidently *beneficent*. The only harm generated is the minimal one of temporary pain from a heel prick. It does not seem rational to say that an exclusion diet is a harm to be avoided when contrasted with a life of handicap.[9] In any event the intention of the doctor is to be beneficent. From a paternalist perspective that is enough.

A contrasting view would be that, in describing this beneficence, we elect as doctors to *prefer* people without mental and physical handicap and in doing so ascribe less value to them. We will consider this point further when considering genetic screening (*see* Chapter 7).

PKU screening follows the principle of *distributive justice* since it is of relatively low cost, includes large numbers of patients, and compares well with the cost of looking after even small numbers of children and adults with learning difficulties. This assumes that there is equality of access to the test, i.e. that there is no variation between districts as to the policy of provision. A centralised healthcare provider such as the NHS is well equipped to achieve this particular aim.

Justice might also require the maintenance of such a screening programme because of the difference in incidence rates quoted above. Areas of the country which have a higher incidence (predominantly Celtic areas) would be more greatly affected by the withdrawal of screening, as more cases would be expected to arise. In a unified healthcare system this would not appear just.

But what of *autonomy*? If we assume that informed consent is an expression of the principle of autonomy, or self-determination, an infant is unable to consent to PKU testing. Therefore the decision devolves to the parents, or to those with parental responsibility. In this context the parents act as proxies in the best interests of the non-autonomous child.

In English law, it is a feature of parental responsibility to have duties to the child, which this sort of decision represents (*see* Chapter 8).[10] In further assessing the best interests of a baby being offered PKU screening, our best decision rests on a balance between the burdens and benefits of the proposed procedure. As described above, the burdens are small: a transient pain as against a lifelong burden.

In most states of the USA, freedom of choice is taken away from the parents by making PKU screening compulsory under law. There is no capacity lawfully to avoid such a test. In effect the parent is denied the option of making an adverse health decision about the child. Put this way, the doctor *qua* state implements a policy of *non-maleficence*.

Using the four principles in this rather brief fashion reassures us that there is a moral case for screening healthy babies for PKU, but some further points, particularly as applied to groups, need more clarification.

The role of utilitarianism

When considering groups, the utilitarian approach seems to apply naturally. It is epitomised in the phrase 'the greatest good for the greatest number'.

Box 4.2   The utilitarian view: a reminder

1   Actions are right if they lead to 'happy' consequences.
2   They are right if those consequences are maximised for as many as possible.
3   In assessing the maximum benefit for a group, each person counts only for one.

Box 4.2 summarises what is known as classical or *act-utilitarianism*.[11] It can be seen at once that the welfare of all is an overriding consideration in moral terms. What might this mean?

First, the will of the majority as expressed by its 'happiness' has moral force. This might be demonstrated by a policy brought about by the NHS, as an expression of the democratic will of the people. That is to say, if the people, via their elected officers, approve and accept a policy of PKU (or any other) screening, it should be determinative.

This idea could be extended, even to overwhelm autonomy. Imagine a situation where screening and treatment for an illness might save money in the long run and that for this to be so the process must involve the whole population at risk, whatever the choice of some members of the population. The utilitarian view would accept the inclusion of a coercive or compulsory element in order to achieve the greater summation of 'happiness' as a result.

Second, what does 'happy' mean? The original utilitarians used this in their writings but over the years critics have suggested modifications to that view. Later philosophers have suggested replacing the word 'happiness' with 'preferences', or have given moral value to the minimisation of 'unhappiness' instead.[12] For example, in the case of PKU there is greater unhappiness attached to the sufferers and their families than would occur if a PKU screening programme were in place.

Third, utilitarianism does not look backward for blame. Actions are deemed right if they lead to positive consequences, however defined. In the case of PKU, an inborn error of metabolism is being searched out by screening and corrected by treatment. Given this positive outcome to treatment, PKU would be considered together with illnesses where, for example, the actions of the patient may have contributed to the illness. The utilitarian would not seek a preference in resource allocation between screening young babies for PKU who are 'blameless' and providing coronary artery bypass grafts for patients who smoke, and thus have contributed to their disease.

Genetic screening

The prenatal period

All GPs know how this issue has moved from the genetic clinic to the consulting room in recent years. GPs and other primary care staff discuss with patients such matters as prenatal screening, where the only option is consideration of termination of pregnancy or, increasingly, preconceptual identification of disease. Sophisticated evaluation of risk lies within the province of the genetic counsellor, but primary care deals with individuals from the perspective of previous knowledge of the patient. Such knowledge could help people make better informed decisions.

The key ethical difference between decisions in this area and other decisions is that they affect the next generation in fundamental ways. We will use the term prenatal to describe the screening of at-risk populations before an affected child is born. Prenatal screening can be undertaken in at-risk populations for disorders like Down's syndrome and selective termination of pregnancy can be considered.

In this way screening poses an awkward moral dilemma for all concerned, which is not made any easier for the GP when counselling the mother. A doctor who persuades a pregnant woman into screening runs the risk of being labelled coercive, as does one who persuades into termination of pregnancy. A better situation prevails when a doctor *fosters autonomy* in his patient; where the doctor's intervention brings about the conditions wherein a patient can make a free and uncoerced choice. Such a consultation would need to address the ideas, concerns and expectations of the patient.

Future generations

Some serious genetic conditions only develop in later life after a period unburdened by symptoms. Genetic screening for these late onset conditions can be regarded rather differently from those already discussed, where the responsibility for making decisions about genetic disease rests on those with parental responsibility. In the case of late onset disease such decisions might be diffused around the family, remembering that the disease could be passed on to the next generation before, or in spite of, identification.

Astrid consults her GP one evening. She is a 25-year-old postgraduate student and has been involved in a population study conducted at her university. She volunteered for a screening test evaluation for risks of Alzheimer's disease and turned out to have a gene associated with an increased risk of Alzheimer's. The exact inheritance mode was as yet undetermined but some additional risk to her children of developing Alzheimer's was inevitable in their lifetime.

She lives with Carl, a City analyst, and they had plans to start a family the next year. Terribly upset at this news, she asked for some advice, including requesting that he inform her sister Dilly, who is also a registered patient.

Pandora's box has been opened by Astrid's participation in this screening experiment. The GP would no doubt wonder how she got involved. The study does not accord with some of the WHO principles listed in Box 4.1. Alzheimer's disease, though common and significantly disabling, has no accepted treatment as yet, and there is no policy which indicates who should be offered the various new experimental treatments. But apparently this is a research project, and the WHO principles apply to established screening processes on offer to all. Clearly as knowledge advances, GPs are going to find themselves in this position more and more in years to come.[13]

What ought the GP do? Of what ethical perspectives should he be aware?

Obviously the GP will need to devote time to listening to all of Astrid's concerns about this new risk and the effect on her future family. He will enquire about her existing family members, and the presence of Alzheimer's disease and other pathology. He might contact the research institute involved for more information, and even question the ethical approval for the study. More than anything else he will support Astrid and Carl through this period.[14]

He might wonder whether this research was *beneficent*. Astrid has been given information about her future which, which is uncertain, but carries the threat of a serious illness. From a general uncertainty about the risk of future illness which we all carry, she is now in what could be termed a specific uncertainty. Furthermore, the threat is of an illness which, rather than making her physically infirm, will undermine her personality, make her dependent on others and probably shorten her life. She does not know how Carl will react to this news of possible future events. Will he remain with her, or want them to bear children together?

What was the quality of consent that Astrid gave to this research? Was she in a position to know all of these possibilities before she took the test? What matters here is another of the components of *autonomy*, that of understanding. Had Astrid made a fully informed consent to the test, then that aspect of autonomy would have been fulfilled. The question remains as to how fully informed one can be in such a situation.

Information, in this context, can span a variety of different meanings, from what the subject might want to know (as in questions asked) to a long exposition on genetic theory and Alzheimer's disease. Whatever the research body had done, Astrid's GP might well take the view that part of his obligation to Astrid was to go back over this ground and check her understanding, appropriate to her new knowledge. He might also wonder whether it was in her best interests to know of her personal results, rather than the researchers holding anonymised information, as is currently the case in other areas.[15]

The role of rights theory

This sort of issue could be addressed under the 'right to know' heading. Anonymised screening where subjects are tested and not informed of the results is well established, though it is the subject of recent challenge.[15] Antenatal screening for human immunodeficiency virus (HIV) has been carried out on this basis for some years to establish population parameters and to plan for the future. The argument against withholding adverse information in this area is essentially one based on *rights*.

> Does Dilly have a right to know that an adverse family history that might affect her and her children has been identified in her sister?

Box 4.3   Rights theory: a reminder

- Rights are justified claims on others
- Rights imply obligations on others
- Legal rights are not necessarily moral rights
- Rights can be negative as well as positive

To put it another way, might Dilly have a right *not* to know about this information? It can be argued that she must be told for all sorts of reasons. She cannot plan her life without knowing of a severe risk to its quality and length, even though the risk is as yet unquantifiable. This would represent the justification for the claim on Astrid for information. If a right to such information exists, a duty is created on those concerned to give it to her. It is a *positive* right to important facts. By contrast a right not to know, if present, is a *negative* right not to be interfered with. That interference could take the form of a species of social discrimination: not being able to be employed, get insurance or adopt, for example.[16]

If it is acknowledged that Dilly should be told of her risk, who should tell her? Astrid is asking that her GP should do this for her, and perhaps, when the immediate dust has settled, this might be for the best. The GP might be familiar with the opinion of the Nuffield Council of Bioethics that has stated that genetic information to third parties is best communicated by family members or doctors if empowered to do so.[17] There is considerable force in the argument that if requested to do so he should go along with Astrid's wishes, assuming that he sees it to be in her best interests, and accepts Dilly's right to be so informed.[18]

The value of persons

The discussion so far has focused on the information aspect of this case. There is a more fundamental issue at stake, which is the idea of *value* mentioned above. Astrid and Carl may elect not to have children because of the risk to them from a susceptibility to Alzheimer's in later life. In doing so, they remove from the population, in advance, people who might have been there, because of an affliction of later life. Also the earlier life from infancy to the onset of the disease is removed as well. Astrid might argue that this view is right because she herself bears such a risk, which if it comes about will require care from her children which they may not be able to provide. The screening test has given her the ability to mould the population of the future.

In doing so, less value is accorded to those who have a future chance of disease. This contrasts with the problem in a late onset disease like Huntingdon's chorea where the Mendelian inheritance pattern offers families a more mathematically predictable course of events. But in that disorder too, a decision to avoid the birth of a potentially affected person is to say that the presymptomatic phase of life is valued less than the sum of that period and the symptomatic phase together. That is an uncomfortable notion for those who would hold that all human life has equal value. It is a feature of this case that Alzheimer's disease is not easily amenable to treatment. This might change, of course, but would it change the ethics underpinning the decisions?

An example: hereditary haemochromatosis (HH)

This is a common problem (1 in 300 in Australia) and can be contrasted with cystic fibrosis (CF), for example (1 in 2500). Identification of these patients by screening will prevent disease, as in the case of PKU. Clinical manifestation of the disease occurs in homozygotes; heterozygotes suffer little if any clinical disorder, but identifying them by screening raises different problems. Allen and Williamson[19] make a strong case for screening young adults for this common disease to avoid personal cost: regular venesection prevents most manifestations of serious illness.

This situation is where the disease being identified might be treatable, or where timely measures can be taken to prevent the disease progressing – like PKU. A public health decision is needed which offers population screening in definable and treatable disease that follows a Mendelian genetic pattern. The possibility arises of 'breeding out' the disease by counselling heterozygous couples or selectively terminating affected pregnancies. It could be argued, as Allen and Williamson do, that this is not appropriate because affected children can be treated with great effect.

Screening and eugenics

Espousing the eradication of a disease like HH, or indeed other similarly inherited diseases like CF, requires us to accept that moulding the population is a good thing. It might be cost-effective: a recent study of CF suggested it might be so,[20] but there are dangers. It should be noted that any cost-effectiveness is a 'good' to the rest of the population: we save money by the avoidance of costs in care of CF patients and so more is available for the rest of us. It is a clearly utilitarian view demonstrated by the maximisation of benefit to the greatest number.[21]

The greater difficulty is to accept that eugenic manipulation is a reasonable aim: Glover has posed the question:

What sort of people should there be?[22]

Many will recoil intuitively from such a prospect, but further consideration will suggest reasons for its proposition.

First, we all seek to better our children's prospects by nurturing, leading, educating and other means. The goal, realised to a greater or lesser extent, is for them to reach their potential and lead happy lives. Caplan even argues a similarity, on the grounds of subjectivity, between the religious values that are handed to children and the potential genetic endowments.[23]

> Why should this process not begin prenatally?

Second, it is a reasonable extension of the doctor's duty to prevent disease and to avoid preventable genetically determined disease. Population screening of this type is but the first step to achieving this end.

Third, we select our children already, at least in part, by the procreative partners we choose. Culture, race and education are all relevant to this.

> Could the practice of eugenics be a reasonable extension of genetic screening?

Other than intuitive recoil, what might be the arguments against such a practice? Here the discussion becomes inevitably less biological and more social. Genetic screening of populations, with population manipulation as a consequence, would render people less varied and diverse. Certainly we might have less genetically determined diseases, but at the same time we might see the allocation of less value to people who are afflicted: that is to say, genetically disadvantaged. In an environment of scarce resources, a pressure might come from planners to coercively test people for genetic disease with the aim of its eradication.

Resistance to a programme of screening for sickle cell disease and trait has been identified on the grounds of stigmatisation because of its greater prevalence in black populations, with hinting at race discrimination as an association.[24] Practical problems also arise as to the way such populations might be identified.[25] Yet in the case of thalassaemia – another recessively inherited haemoglobinopathy – there are now almost no new births of affected babies in Cyprus, where previously there was a high incidence. This has been brought about by a combination of an intensive education campaign and screening. Gill and Modell note that this is not the case in the UK for Asian populations, though it is for Cypriot ones, and advance practical solutions to this state of affairs.[26] They suggest that primary care is the best place for carrier screening to be done so as to reduce the discrepancy in information provision that underlies the birth of new thalassaemics to mainly Asians in the UK. In doing so, populations are moulded and individual harms reduced.

Harms in screening

Beneficence and non-maleficence

The principle of non-maleficence states that doctors are required not to harm their patients. At first sight, it seems that it is difficult to harm people when considering a process that seeks out disease in order to eliminate or prevent it. But it is possible to identify harms here, which may outweigh the benefits of screening.

The first harm has already been mentioned: the anxiety and worry related to the process and results of screening examinations.[14,27] It is prudent to remember screened people are well people who only contract in as a result of medical action. Even when patients request screening procedures following publicly available health information the original cue is generally research-based, although this may sometimes be of dubious quality.

Another harm is more subtle and is related to the tendency of screening procedures to aim primarily at human longevity. Herman[28] describes a culture of 'cholesterol awareness' achieving only an extra 18 months of life per person for members of a high-risk group. Overall, people got three extra weeks of life on average. Whilst this may be fine as far as it goes, that extra span is added onto the end of life, where faculties and quality of life may be less than at a younger age. If this evidence is duplicated, the question needs to be asked whether all this screening, prevention and work is worth the effort for such a modest gain.

Herman's argument asks us to consider whether screening should work to improve the years we have rather than necessarily adding to them. An extension of this argument is that an environment of medicalisation of everyday life is created, which ultimately becomes coercive, and that this is harmful to individual decision making and happiness. It is a short step from what is described as 'coercive healthism'[29] to legitimising a duty to oneself to health improvement. When doctors think this way then patients do not always appreciate it.[30]

This kind of discussion is interesting because it illuminates an aspect of autonomy often overlooked: that of *controlling influences*. Briefly what is involved here is that we can only be said to make autonomous decisions when there are no external controlling influences that overly guide, or coerce, behaviour. These authors claim that an environment of what is tantamount to coercion is created by doctors and others who look more to the health of populations than individuals.

They also argue that doctors' roles should be concerned with the relief of suffering by patients rather than 'social' engineering. The roots of this argument lie in a conception of liberty as a 'negative' right to not be interfered with, as long as no harm comes to others, and described in the nineteenth century by John Stuart Mill.

Limits to utilitarianism

Ethics, being concerned with defining the 'right' action, must also be concerned with assessing 'rightness'; harms and benefits are part of this equation. But another view of how this may be assessed comes from proposals to screen for *Chlamydia trachomatis* in asymptomatic women. The prize is 30 000 fewer cases of pelvic inflammatory disease (PID) over five years in the UK.

From the utilitarian perspective this is faultless:

- less unhappiness would occur, exemplified by PID and its consequences
- more happiness would occur as there would be more PID free women and less reduced fertility thereafter
- no discussions would be necessary about how the chlamydia infection arose[31]
- the eventual eradication of chlamydia in the population would clearly be a positive outcome
- the popularity of screening validates its 'rightness' on democratic grounds.

But as Duncan and Hart note, it is not that simple.[32] There is potential harm that may not be outweighed by the above observations, though it is of subtler dimension. *Inter alia*, they draw attention to the implicit sexual surveillance taking place in the screened population and the relative exclusion of men from taking responsibility for chlamydia transmission. These kinds of more subtle harms are difficult to integrate into the utilitarian calculus of positives and negatives. While it is naturally part of the utilitarian approach to consider populations, this theory has limits in assessing some screening programmes.

It has been said that all public health measures are utilitarian in flavour, but perhaps what we should envisage are *deontological constraints* upon them or limitations based upon respect for persons. To take the above example, a constraint on a publicly funded chlamydia screening programme as described might be to allow for testing of men too, or a synchronous health education campaign for all, rather than a mechanistic testing of women of the target group. In this way, ethical justification for the process is more easily argued.

Financial implications

A potential ethical problem arises where there is a covert financial inducement for screening. The offer of a 'free' health check may be attractive to many asymptomatic apparently healthy individuals. This may be funded by the employer at no cost to the employee, who will then be given a print-out of the results of the various tests performed.

A COMPANY AND CO.

Personnel Dept

As a valued employee, your health matters to us.

Keep healthy and have a free check by our team of expert doctors after work.

They will look for early signs of illness so you can sort them out straight away!

On the face of it, A Company and Co. is behaving with great altruism in funding free health checks for their employees.[33]

If the health check on offer provides for the review of the risk factors of the employee by a doctor or nurse, then that is probably true: they are functioning as a source of health advice and information which may empower the employee to improve their health (with the caveats mentioned above). If the company doctor or some such delegated doctor then runs a series of expensive tests to 'look out for early signs of illness' it could become less so. In asymptomatic patients, the pick up rate for abnormalities that are significant is generally low; the company is investing a substantial amount to little obvious beneficial effect.

Contrast this with the known determinants of health, which comprise diet, smoking, housing and poverty. It sits ill with the aim of health prevention policy to accord these factors less importance than a screening test for, say, liver function. In the end the moral justification should rest on the practical justification exemplified by, for example, the WHO criteria (*see* Box 4.1).[34]

Risk

Risk has already been mentioned in this chapter. It is pertinent to examine this in more detail at this point. The ultimate aim of screening is to reduce risks of illness to individuals and to populations. We can think of this in several ways.

Risk magnitude is generally taken to mean the gravity of the problem of which one takes a risk. Clearly Alzheimer's disease is a graver risk than, say, a penicillin rash.

Absolute risk defines the chances of an event occurring, and in the medical context is equivalent to incidence. This can be personalised, for example the risk of a major cardiac event occurring in a male smoker of 60 years with borderline lipids and borderline high blood pressure is 30%.[35] Relative risk would merely indicate how much more likely he is to get his event than, say, a non-smoker. It has been said that policy decisions should only be made on assessments of absolute risk.[36]

Probability lies at the heart of risk. It is an expression of the likelihood of an adverse event occurring, or indeed any event, though it seems perverse in a medical context to talk of the risks of a positive event. Doctors are fond of mathematical risk formulations, probably because such concrete figures have the patina of science. How much this means to patients is open to question and recalls again the discussion of how informed is informed. Slaytor and Ward, for example, describe selective risk description in pamphlets about mammography to encourage take up of the service.[37] By implication this will only occur where patients lack a sophisticated understanding of risk. Moreover, if the population of the UK really understood how weak the chances of winning, say, the National Lottery were, would they spend as much on it as they do?[38] Perhaps we will do better by talking of the benefits and burdens of a particular treatment, or non-treatment, and the risks of either.

What clouds doctors' and patients' understanding of risk is the presence of uncertainty. Astrid had knowledge of an increased risk, only a statistical notion, but no idea of whether she would lie in the affected group or not. Perhaps she would not. What she had been given was an increased but uncertain chance of a nasty disease. It could be argued that the uncertainty is reason enough not to inform her of the result, as the harm flows directly from the uncertainty as much as the illness. When the future is only a matter of conjecture, as in this case, no further action should be taken. In Astrid's case that would be a paternalist view needing strong justification.

From the utilitarian perspective, risks need to be incorporated into the equation of negatives and positives that determine moral value. Reigelbaum has suggested a scheme for assessing the value of a treatment to an individual within a scarce resource environment based on a sum of probability of benefit and utility to that individual, expressed mathematically.[39] In this way priorities can be set between individuals with some ethical justification.

It is difficult to harmonise rule-based ethics with the notion of risk. Rules do not allow for uncertainty. For example, English statute law allows abortion if:

> ... there is a substantial risk that if the child were born it would suffer from such physical or mental abnormalities as to be seriously handicapped[40]

Or to paraphrase, the chances of being born seriously handicapped allow for termination of the pregnancy, where risk is determinative. Those who hold to the sanctity of life doctrine and cannot allow destruction of life (defined from conception onward) can allow no leeway for risk of handicap or anything else.

Cervical screening revisited

This chapter concludes with another look at cervical screening, which forms such a large part of the work of the primary healthcare team. As has been said, this intervention is conducted on about four million women in the UK each year, with the aim of reducing the incidence and mortality of invasive cervical cancer. From the evidence there seems to be some agreement about a positive effect globally,[41] but the extent of this is unclear, and the downside is not fully evaluated. For example, a high false-positive rate gives rise to over-investigation and engenders undue anxiety in the patient.[42] All this arises from potentially conflicting empirical evidence.

But there are additional moral issues too. Foster and Anderson draw our attention to a problem peculiar to the UK. Here, GPs are 'fined'; that is to say, their income is reduced if they do not manage to screen a percentage of the target population of women each quarter of the year. Could this have the effect of encouraging GPs and their staff to exert pressure on women to get their cervical smears done where the benefit to the population is empirically dubious?[43] If women are being screened under a coercive regime (evidenced by the GP pay arrangements and a strong public health campaign) the ethical principles of respect for persons and individual autonomy are undermined. They suggest that a more ethically sound basis for such screening would be based on considerably more information being given to patients. A personal risk assessment for each woman would be needed, with GPs encouraging screening only when based on this assessment. This would answer the requirement for a patient to be fully informed in order to make an autonomous decision whether or not to accept cervical screening. We could argue that the necessity for GPs to achieve a certain target in order to attract a fee for service is inconsistent with respect for persons.[44]

The notion of personal risk with regard to screening is of particular interest as there is some evidence that the cervical screening programme would be more productive if targeted in some way – perhaps to high-risk groups. This proposal moves the aim of such screening away from the good of the community as a whole to that of the person in particular.

Box 4.4   Risk factors in cervical cancer[45]

Human papilloma virus contact
Low age of first intercourse
Low socioeconomic group
Oral contraception
Smoking
Penile cancer
Chlamydia trachomatis

There are dangers in identifying specific groups for screening. As we have seen, a proposed screening programme for chlamydia infection exposes potential harms which will need to be dealt with sensitively. All of these risk factors listed in Box 4.4 share that danger. It is also important to note that, were a targeted screening system put in hand, some unscreened 'low-risk' women would still develop their cervical cancers, despite paying through taxation for a service to everyone: how can priorities be set? (*See* Chapter 10.)

A US case resulted in a doctor being held in negligence for not warning a patient of the consequences of declining a cervical smear test. She died of cervical cancer. The judges in majority held that the doctor had a duty to warn her of the risks of *not* having a screening test. Interestingly, the judge who dissented acknowledged that if doctors had such a duty they would spend all their time teaching people about medical science, as part of pre-test counselling, rather than practising medicine, with consequent administrative and financial problems.[46] There is no English law on this as yet, but the underlying principles are of interest. The case lends weight to the proposal that in order to be ethically sound, screening procedures ought to be accompanied by more individualised information than at present.

Conclusion

This chapter has reviewed the reasons to screen populations from the moral as well as the practical point of view. A tacit assumption underlying screening is that where populations are benefited, as a matter of public health or health improvement, so are individuals. We have argued that this is not necessarily the case. GPs have duties to individuals but also to populations and screening is one part of this duty. The balance between harm and benefit in the screening process is difficult to achieve; it is made even more difficult on occasions by the obligation to implement national policies. The complexity of assessing the moral worth of screening is illustrated by any of the examples that have been mentioned in this chapter. Finally, the following questions need consideration when assessing the moral worth of screening procedures.

- Do the benefits of a system outweigh the harms?
- Does the intention to benefit the public good take account of individuals' choices?
- Are such choices adequately informed?
- What sort of populations do we want as a result of screening?
- How do we balance cost of prevention against treatment?
- Whom do we screen?

References and notes

1   Koestler A (1939) *The Gladiators.* Hutchinson, Danube edition. (A tale of Spartacus.)

2   The Terms of Service of GPs paras 14 (1) and 14 (2) require a GP to write to a new patient offering participation in a registration examination, which must include these measurements. Paras 23 (1–5) defines the payment for this task in *Statement of Fees and Allowances* (1996), commonly known as the 'Red Book'.

3   Tudor Hart avers a moral obligation, if not a legal one, on the part of GPs to screen adults 5 yearly for raised BP to prevent the tragedy of vascular disease. *See* Hart T (1992). In:C Hart and P Burke (eds) *Screening and Surveillance in General Practice.* Churchill Livingstone, Edinburgh.

4   Wilson JNG and Jungner G (1968) *Principles and Practice of Screening for Disease.* World Health Organization.

5   Radford M (1999) Early diagnosis of child cancer. *Practitioner.* **243**: 664–70.

6   See NHSCSP (1999) *Cervical Screening – a pocket guide,* essentially a guide for patients. Also a discussion of the screening and mortality question in Quinn *et al.* (1999) UK Ass. of Cancer Registries. *BMJ* **318**: 904–8 3rd April and comment by several writers *BMJ.* **318**: 642–3 4th Sept.

7   For a summary of this position, see Fowler G, Gray M and Anderson P (eds). *Prevention in General Practice* (2e). Ch. 10, p. 122 *et seq.*

8   *The Times.* **9 March 2000,** p. 12.

9   A recent study of children in the second year of life found that a thumb prick screening test for anaemia was 'acceptable' in the terms researched, which was in terms of distress to the child, perhaps validating the WHO criterion above. Goodhart C and Logan S (1999) Acceptability of screening young children for anaemia. *Br J Gen Pract.* **49**: 907–8.

10   That parental 'rights' over children are flowing from duties to them is fully expounded by Lord Scarman in Gillick v West Norfolk and Wisbech Area Health Authority (1986) *AC*: 112.

11   A recommended account of this and other moral theories can be found in Rachels J (1994) *The Elements of Moral Philosophy.* McGraw Hill International Edition.

12   Utilitarianism as the minimisation of unhappiness or harms is known as *negative utilitarianism* in philosophical writings. For the analysis of happiness and preference *see* Ayer AJ (1990) Happiness as satisfaction of desires. In: J Glover (ed.) *Utilitarianism and its Critics.* Macmillan, Basingstoke.

13   Explicitly acknowledged in Advisory Committee on Genetic Testing (1998) *Report on Genetic Testing for Late Onset Disorders.* Health Depts. of UK.

14 Marteau TM and Croyle RT (1998) Psychological responses to genetic testing. *BMJ* 316: 693–6.

15 de Zulueta P (2000) The ethics of anonymised HIV testing of pregnant women: a reappraisal. *J Med Ethics.* 26: 16–21. This article is followed by a commentary and reply, which further illuminate the topic.

16 For a full discussion of this issue *see* Wilke JTR (1998) Late onset genetic disease: where ignorance is bliss, is it folly to inform relatives? *BMJ.* 317: 744–7.

17 This was the position in 1993. *See* Nuffield Council on Bioethics (London) *Genetic Screening: Ethical Issues.* Also supported in 1998.

18 Takala T and Gylling HA (2000) Who should know about our genetic makeup and why? *J Med Ethics.* 26: 171–4. The authors conclude no one is bound or entitled to genetic knowledge.

19 Allen K and Williamson R (1999) Should we test everyone for haemochromatosis? *J Med Ethics.* 25: 209–14.

20 Cuckle HS, Richardson GA, Sheldon TA and Quirke P (1995) Cost effectiveness of antenatal screening for cystic fibrosis. *BMJ.* 311: 1460. A cost per affected pregnancy is determined to inform healthcare purchasing policy.

21 In the case of HH there is an advantage to the illness in one small sense. Apparently the iron overload is of benefit in one stage of life, in pregnancy. Illnesses are not always universally negative things.

22 Glover J (1977) *What Sort of People Should There Be?* Penguin, London.

23 Caplan AL, McGhee G and Magnus D (1999) What is immoral about eugenics? *BMJ.* 319: 1284–5.

24 Sickle cell carriers in the US were refused health insurance and had difficulties with adoption. Such discrimination is now illegal there, but not in the UK. *See* Laird L, Dezateux C and Anionwuru EN (1996) Neonatal screening for SC disorders: what about the carrier infant? *BMJ.* 313: 407–11.

25 Streetly A (2000) National screening policy for sickle cell disease and thalassaemia major for the UK. *BMJ.* 320: 1353–4.

26 Gill PS and Modell B (1998) Thalassaemia in Britain: a tale of two communities. *BMJ.* 317: 761–2.

27 Mayou R (1996) Screening in primary care: pointers for further research. *B J Gen Pract.* **Oct**: 567–8.

28 Herman J (1996) The ethics of prevention: old twists and new. *Br J Gen Pract.* **46**: 547–9.

29 Skrabanek P (1994) *The Death of Humane Medicine.* Social Affairs Unit, London.

30 A Norwegian study described the poor satisfaction of patients with exhortations of doctors to reduce coronary risk as against a patient centred approach. *See* Maeland E *et al.* (1996) Lifestyle interventions in general

practice: effects on psychological well being and patient satisfaction. *Quality of Life Research.* **5**: 348–54.

31 Patients and their partners are usually very concerned about the source of their sexually transmitted disease when it is diagnosed – who is to 'blame'?

32 Duncan B and Hart G (1999) Sexuality and health: the hidden costs of screening for *Chlamydia trachomatis*. *BMJ*. **318**: 931–3.

33 Although we note that it takes place 'after work' and not in company time.

34 Counter-arguments but no evidence are to be found in Gibson K (1999) Private health screening. *B J Gen Pract*. **48**: 1703.

35 Jackson R (2000) Guidelines on preventing cardiovascular disease in clinical practice. *BMJ*. **320**: 659–61.

36 Rose G (1991) Environmental health: prospects and problems. *J R Coll Physicians Lond*. **25**: 48–52.

37 Slaytor EK and Ward JE (1998) How risks of breast cancer and benefits of screening are communicated to women: analysis of 58 pamphlets. *BMJ*. **317**: 263–4.

38 Said to be 1 in 14 000 000. This theme is further developed in Chapter 6.

39 Reigelbaum R (1994) *The Measures of Medicine*. Blackwell, Oxford, Ch. 5.

40 S1(1)d Abortion Act 1967 (modified by Human Embryology and Fertilisation Act 1990). This Act provides a defence to the charge of procuring a miscarriage as under the Offences against the Person Act 1861.

41 Fylan F (1998) Screening for cervical cancer: a review of women's attitudes, knowledge and behaviour. *Br J Gen Pract*. **48**: 1509–14. The author comments on the success of the programme, and examines non-participation reasons including health belief and information provision.

42 Raffle AE, Alden B and McKenzie EFD (1995) Detection rates for abnormal smears: what are we looking for? *Lancet*. **345**: 1469–73.

43 Foster P and Anderson CM (1998) Reaching targets in the national cervical screening programme: are current practices unethical? *J Med Ethics*. **24**: 151–7.

44 It is interesting to note, in the context of confidentiality, that health authorities require a woman's clinical details before she can be excluded from the GP's target population.

45 The Cochrane Library (1999) *Interventions for Encouraging Sexual Lifestyles and Behaviour Intended to Prevent Cervical Cancer (Protocol for a Cochrane Review)*. Update Software, Oxford.

46 Truman v Thomas (1980) 611 P. 2d 902.

CHAPTER FIVE

Matters of the mind

Summary

This chapter explores some of the ethical problems that arise with patients whose thought processes demonstrate psychiatric or psychological obstructions to their health and well-being.

- What is illness?
- Somatisation
- Unhappy patients
- Problems with substance abuse
- Harm to others: the ethics of intervention
- Harm to self: the ethics of intervention
- Irrational people.

What did it mean to be mad? It meant you had some idea, or some wish so important to you that you were ready to alter your perception of reality, or reality itself, to support it.[1]

Introduction

Strangely enough, literature on the ethics of mental health is not so easy to find, and especially so literature with relevance to primary care.[2] By comparison, there is much written on the legal aspects of mental illness. This chapter will fill some of the gaps by addressing a few specific problems from general practice.

History

Over the centuries, there has been confusion as to the relationship between mental illness and morality itself, let alone the moral aspects of the care of mental illness. Remember that asylums were created as places of care and containment for the behaviourally disordered in the seventeenth and eighteenth centuries in England, and often housed those said to be morally problematic, such as mothers of illegitimate children.[3] Before the scientific era, such disorders were often held to be caused by moral or religious turpitude. Even now, argument can reign over the distinction between 'ill' or 'bad' offenders, a confusion which has moral roots, and which *inter alia* the specialty of forensic psychiatry exists to address.

Of all doctors, those in general practice are most aware of the interplay between physical and mental aspects to illness. Doctors are taught in training to consider all presenting problems in physical, social and psychological terms, almost as a rule of thumb. Various studies of our workload estimate the emotional/behavioural element to be a third to a half of the whole.[4] It is also known that GPs manage 95% of patients with psychiatric disorders.[5]

The GP understands and uses the 'therapeutic relationship' between doctor and patient to aid and guide improvement. The GP's position as the point of first access exposes him or her to raw emotions from life crises of all sorts. McWhinney has even suggested that general practice is the only specialty to:

transcend the dualistic division between mind and body[6]

In conditions that are be termed 'major' psychiatric illnesses, the affective disorders and psychoses, the GP will often have known the evolution of the problem at first hand, and might well be the agent of crisis intervention. The GP will be aware of the impact of these problems on the patient's life and loved ones. Before investigating the ethics of mental illness and health, a short digression into illness models will be helpful.

What is illness?

For a GP, it is tempting to say that illness is whatever the patient brings to the consultation, and avoid further analysis, but this would accommodate many problems that on reflection lie within the domain of another professional's expertise.[7] Much of the GP's work does not involve 'ill' people, however defined: for example, antenatal care, child health surveillance, contraception.[8]

Twelve different illness models that GPs could use to reference their patients' problems have been described by Neighbour; all of these are of great interest when the true reason for a consultation seems obscure and a further analysis is required.[9] Such a framework is necessary to conceptualise illness that takes in the physical, social and psychological aspects yet allow consideration of ethical aspects as well. Most doctors, being raised in the sciences rather than the humanities, will feel at home with a 'biological malfunctioning' model.

Illnesses have specific *causes*: cure must be directed to these causes in order to be successful. This makes sense at a certain level, but seems to break down when one explores it in more detail. For example, impetigo is caused by staphylococci. Why does a particular patient at a particular time, on exposure to staphylococci, get impetigo? There might be a risk factor, like a wound, but then again there might not. The identification of the true causative factor will depend on the limits of empirical observation.[10]

The connection between life events and patterns of illness can certainly be evidenced, though this depends on an adequate classification of these patterns. Craig and Brown, and many others since, demonstrated an association between negative life events and irritable bowel syndrome (IBS).[11] It does not necessarily demonstrate causation. It matters to doctors how illnesses are caused, not just because treatment is determined, but also it defines their attitude to the illnesses and the patients who suffer them.

Given associations like this in IBS, it is not going to be possible to treat it properly (as an exercise in beneficence) without paying attention to such things as the influence of life events on the patient. Beneficence demands skills in both areas, clinical and psychological. IBS and many other illnesses represent an overlap between social and physical processes and blur previously held distinctions

---

Box 5.1   Beneficence – a reminder

The provision of benefits
A moral obligation to provide benefits
Paternalism: where the doctor 'knows best'
But – it may conflict with autonomy

---

between mental and other health problems. Some disorders do seem to be purely of behaviour, mood or thinking. The causative chain is not always easy to discern, perhaps because our level of knowledge is less well developed than in purely physical problems. But the fact remains that, for example, negative life events are also associated with relapses in schizophrenia, implying that we should adopt this biological model of primary mental illness too.[12]

What this conception depends upon is a satisfactory description of each illness that can identify it to practitioners. This aspect, termed *nosology*, is less easy than might at first be thought. Psychiatry has tried to come to grips with this in recent years by the publication of standardised descriptions of illness patterns,[13] but even in physical disorders it can be difficult.[14]

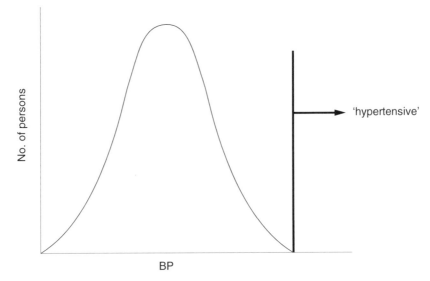

Figure 5.1   Essential hypertension.

Consider essential hypertension, which is defined by reference to outcome (*see* Figure 5.1).

A graph of measurement of blood pressure (BP) plotted against numbers of people of a specific age shows a normal distribution, reflecting frequency. We define the disorder of essential hypertension above a certain point (say 90 mm Hg diastolic) because where the BP is over that point, a significant number of people suffer adverse consequences in time. The further to the right a diastolic BP is, the greater the chance of such consequences. It could almost be said to be a consequentialist definition, shorn of its moral value. However, as we argue throughout this book, shearing away the moral value from any 'clinical' decision or definition is fraught with problems.

> At what point on the normal distribution above is a moral duty to identify and treat raised blood pressure created?

Such a convenient quantitative classification is unavailable in mental health, where a reliance on qualitative description is all there is. Mental illnesses are challenging to categorise; clear biological markers are difficult to identify. Some authors, the 'antipsychiatrists', have been led to deny their existence because they might be considered purely as disorders of behaviour. Szasz, for example, considers psychiatric diagnosis to be a mere stigmatising label, and not representative of 'illness'.[15] Were this really the case, a different task would be apparent for medical ethics. However, given the observations above, it is sensible to use standard ethical frameworks for examination of mental health problems.

Somatisation

Somatisation represents the overlap of physical and mental processes in clinical practice, and is one of the most challenging problems in medical practice. The picture is familiar: a patient presents who is preoccupied with physical symptomatology, looking for an explanation in physical terms, and the doctor is unable to find one.

The example of IBS above represents a form of somatisation, where psychological precipitants are often of great importance to the course of the illness.

Anthony is a 45-year-old fitter. He has suffered recurrent central abdominal pain over 4 years or so, associated with bouts of diarrhoea. In addition, when under stress, he noted limb pains and tiredness, and recurrent headaches. His GP had referred him initially to a gastroenterologist, who performed scans and barium studies without positive findings. His return letter admitted his search for physical pathology had been in vain, suggesting a functional disorder. Anthony had blood tests from time to time and when told all was normal seemed upset and hurt, and asked for further tests. Enquiries about his state of mind were rebuffed. The GP was unsure what to do next.

Anthony's story is typical of patients concerned about physical symptoms of varying degrees of severity but with no clear evidence of physical disease. Despite her best efforts, the doctor is stuck, and does not know how to proceed.

Patients like this have been variously labelled 'difficult', 'heartsink', Briquet's syndrome, somatisers and 'fat file syndrome'. These pejorative terms simply denote the continuing lack of resolution of their symptoms in spite of repeated consultations with GPs and consultants. We could equally well talk of heartsink doctors who are failing the patient in some way if nothing more can be done. A recent review of the philosophical aspects of this area of work identified the nature of the doctor's difficulty as helplessness in the face of a patient's search for a biomedical solution for a spiritual or social problem.[16]

There are valid therapeutic interventions that can be attempted: for example, re-attribution therapy, aimed at identifying underlying stressors and helping patients to make the link from them to their symptoms. Communication between doctor and patient, as always, is pivotal. Two types of explanation about negative test results in patients like Anthony were distinguished in one study. Patients felt 'blamed' or 'empowered' depending on the style of communication. 'Empowering' led to self-management of symptoms.[17]

What are the ethical considerations?

Consider first the duty of the GP. If she colludes with Anthony's desire for further investigations she may be responding to his autonomous wish, but it is hardly in his best interests, since such further tests are probably going to be unrewarding and may carry some risk. A version of paternalism that leads her to desist seems the best way of describing it, if clinically justified. The depth of her duty must be to do her best, rather than make Anthony 'happy' by acceding to his requests for further investigation, or to remove all his unpleasant feelings.[18]

Second, the clinical problem highlights a difference between respecting Anthony's autonomy at the time, and creating autonomy in the future. By behaving in this 'paternalist' fashion now, she might actually respect his future autonomy, when the illness has passed.

There is obviously a tension between these two moral principles so how can it be addressed? Konrad[19] suggests that illness (as exemplified by Anthony's somatisation) is a state of diminished autonomy and thus the sick actually require paternalistic treatment limited to maximising the patient's autonomy at the conclusion of treatment. One could consider this aspect under the 'controlling influences' component of autonomy.

Pellegrino[20] puts things a little stronger, arguing that illness is an assault on our being (an ontological assault) which impedes our choices and actions and compromises our freedoms. He quotes Hippocrates from *On Diseases* as follows:

> If the physician is to help, his relationship to the patient must be that of the person in command to one who obeys

which sounds archaic in the twenty-first century, but Pellegrino sees it as a hint at justification for occasional paternalism in practice. If this sort of maxim is followed, then Anthony should obey his GP because she knows what is best, and she cannot help without his obedience. It is supported by O'Neill's suggestion that:

> patients *standardly* have reduced cognitive and volitional capacities[21]

On this analysis, the ruthless search for organic pathology in this sort of patient could be termed maleficent. It could well offend the principle of justice too, since healthcare resources would be ineffectively and inappropriately consumed by Anthony and his doctor together.

Another insight comes from Toon[22] who considers virtue ethics in the context of general practice. He argues that some problems, of which care of somatisers would be a good example, offer a particular challenge to the doctor. Work with these patients requires the virtues of moral courage and fortitude in the doctor. Many other conditions might require similar virtues. Whether this can be acquired, or is intrinsic to the practitioner, would be another area of discussion.

Unhappy patients

As suggested above, many patients present to the GP with physical symptoms without any physical explanation for them, but another large group present as unhappy or 'depressed'. Patients often describe their problems in a confusing way, demonstrating to the listener the internal confusion that they are feeling.[23] Diagnostic criteria are difficult to apply. How are we to proceed?[24]

Briony was under pressure at work. She was asked to do more and more tasks at her job in publishing, and found herself staying late at the office and rushing back to pick her children up from a child minder. She had to attend weekend conferences and missed her family and friends, as well as her children, as a consequence. She began to sleep badly and became snappy with all who met her, She spent time in the toilet at work sobbing.

Becoming like this prompted her to see her GP for advice. He gave her some time to talk of her feelings and he asked further questions about her lifestyle, upbringing and marriage.

He reflected on how else he might assist.

The clinical problem is not easy. GPs take full histories to clarify feelings and emotions and the personal problems currently at issue. There may be previous knowledge of the patient and their family, job and the rest of the background. Diagnostic rating scales such as the Beck's inventory or the Hamilton Rating Scale might aid a classi-fication of the patients' problems in formal psychiatric terms.[25]

Having done this, the GP will try and tackle the problem by talk-ing, treating with drugs, or asking for specialist help. All this approx-imates to the standard 'medical model' view of these interactions. There are other models too numerous to go into here, so for the moment we will assume the standard model as described for a further analysis.

On a continuum between mild unhappiness or anxiety and psychotic depression, where is Briony's 'illness'? Does it matter? When is it right to embark on pharmacological treatment?

One answer to this latter question is circular. Ashton memorably described:

> ... a tendency to give patients with emotional disturbance a hard psychiatric label to justify the use of a psychotropic drug.[26]

This implies, for example, that in some cases patients need a diag-nosis of depression in order to 'earn' their antidepressant. Put more forcefully, the diagnosis could be an 'antidepressant responsive dis-order' in anticipation of a prescription. This is not just to say that the cart is preceding the horse but perhaps that there is more power exercised by the makers of psychotropic medications than thought generally.[27]

If we accept that certain life events like work stress or unemploy-ment are causative, or at least associative, in affective disorders of this type, then 'treatment' by drugs, in the long run, seems inap-propriate compared to social action to ameliorate this causative factor. There is a powerful moral argument to reshape social policy as a preventive measure in a way that fosters mental and emotional health.[28]

Briony's case history raises some profound questions about a GP's role. He might conceptualise the problem clinically and conclude Briony is depressed, recommending treatment along these lines: antidepressants and supportive therapy. On the other hand, he might switch out of a medical role to a more patient-oriented one, giving or referring for formal counselling. Arguably any of these roles fulfils the requirement to be *beneficent,* to do Briony some good and to alleviate her distress.[29]

However, a big problem appears to be out of his control – the overwhelming management under which Briony labours, and over which she herself has little control. No doubt clarification of this aspect of the problem will be part of the support he can offer her. It could be argued that any 'treatment' for her 'illness' is covering over a deeper problem arising out of adverse work conditions and perhaps the GP should be addressing the company directly. That might seem inconsistent with what is generally thought of as a GP's role, but has some force of logic. Why, after all, should psychotropic drugs cover for bad work practices? This approach has all sorts of problems such as confidentiality, pride and legal liability, but has some echoes of the argument advanced above.

There is an analogy with the treatment of patients with asthma who smoke. One clinical argument says that the medical treatment of such patients is useless since the smoking subverts attempts at pharmacological control of illness. But most, if not all, GPs continue to try and respond to the 'need' of smokers with asthma by continuing to prescribe suitable inhalers. Clearly this arises from a notion of beneficence. It could also be described as a doctor accommodating a patient's adverse health practices. Perhaps an old-fashioned exhortation to stop smoking, forcefully backed up by a refusal to prescribe without such action, may be more productive in the long run, albeit by coercive paternalism. The ultimate aim would be the provision of benefit in the sense of short- and long-term health. Benefit is not necessarily only about health, defined in bio-medical terms, as we shall see below.[30] This demonstrates that situations where external events are potentially modifiable affect the ethics of a particular clinical problem.

Problems with substance abuse

Many of us take substances which interfere with our health. The list is potentially endless, and the unifying feature, it is said, is the harm that they do to us. However, consider this a little deeper. First, as is related elsewhere, do we have a duty to do the best for ourselves, such that this duty requires us to bear the consequences of indulging in dangerous drug taking? That might be the basis of the refusal, or difficulty, of getting medical help with the problem.

Second, the definitions of harm are rather elastic. Smoking seems to be universally harmful as there are no benefits to it, other than perhaps the transient pleasurable sensation at first 'drag' which most smokers and ex-smokers will cheerfully report. That said, part of the habituation of cigarette smoking consists for some people in its assistance with life's everyday stresses. If healthcare professionals accept a consistency of harm from smoking, or an overall harm over benefit, they ought to work towards its eradication.

But what of alcohol? The 'U-shaped curve' of alcohol mortality is now well known.[31] In brief, teetotallers have an excess all-cause mortality over those who drink around 8–10 units of alcohol per week, but increasing levels of usage above this level have the effect of increasing mortality. Interestingly enough this phenomenon was confirmed in a prospective study of doctors.[32] Morally speaking, it could be advocated that GPs ought to be pointing this out to patients; but does the observed U-shaped curve confer a duty on patients to drink a little alcohol each week?

It seems risible for a GP to be in the position of persuading a temperate person to consume small quantities of alcohol regularly to preserve health. To accept a moral course for this is to accept there is a duty of self-preservation, but also that the care of this particular patient at this particular time carries a reciprocal duty on the part of the GP.

The large population-based studies referred to above reflect the state of knowledge at the time. They have the potential of informing public policy making, but the extension of the general to the particular in this case seems illogical. It is really a version of the philosophical fallacy that it is not right to construct what one *ought* to do from what *is*. The fact of the U-shaped curve, as determined by observation, cannot determine individual behaviour duties. By extension, if a patient lies at the extreme right of the curve and drinks heavily, that is not necessarily morally wrong and therefore we as doctors cannot fence ourselves off from the care of such persons. Whether we can *preferentially* allocate resources in a way that disadvantages people on the right of the curve is a different argument (*see* Chapter 10). And is self-inflicted harm necessarily wrong?

Third, what of the issue of responsibility? Consider this case.

Chris had just moved to the practice area of a suburban GP. At his first appointment, he told her of his use of heroin over some years. He had several criminal convictions for drug-related offences. He said he was hepatitis C positive and HIV negative. He had just moved in with a local girlfriend, and was keen to try and stop his habit. He asked for a methadone prescription and when she hesitated about this, said he'd be happy with diazepam only to keep him calm, but his usual dose was 40 mg per day. Her further hesitation caused him to get agitated. He said that if she would not prescribe he'd have to get some 'gear' from the street.

Let us deal with one issue first. The GP has a professional duty to Chris as a registered patient. She cannot evade doing something for Chris even if she wants to because of his way of life. The UK General Medical Council puts it most strongly. In doing so, the moral rule founded on a conception of a doctor's duty is elevated to a binding professional guideline.

> You must not deny or delay investigation or treatment because you believe that the patient's actions or lifestyle may have contributed to their condition.[33]

That said, it is difficult to conceive of any GP washing her hands of patients like Chris any more, though negative attitudes among health professionals do remain towards drug abusers.[34] In any event, the duty at law should be added to the moral and professional duties already mentioned. The discussion therefore moves to the scope of the doctor's duty and what that might mean (*see* Chapter 2).

What part does beneficence play in the consultation with Chris?

Chris takes drugs to maintain some sort of equilibrium in his life yet with a degree of addiction. We know that if he is refused there will be drug supply 'on the street', as he puts it, or ensuing criminal activity.

There are certainly moral reasons with a utilitarian base for accepting his requests for drugs on medical prescription, reasons which spring from the possible consequences of non-prescription.

The evidence for them is demonstrated in a study showing that GP care of heroin addicted patients reduced imprisonment and criminal conviction.[35] Notice that some of these reasons flow from the reduction of harms to other people beside the patient, such that the impetus to treat Chris is at least partially for the good of others. This aspect is typical of the utilitarian view, aiming towards 'the greatest good to the greatest number'.

Box 5.2   Reasons for doctors to supply addictive drugs

Minimisation of harms
Maintenance of *status quo*
Prevention of harm to others: family
Prevention of harm to others: criminality
Reducing the illicit market
Aiming for future drug-free existence

A deontological argument supporting such a decision seems to be a version of respect for autonomy; Chris requests opiates or other drugs and the GP carries out his wish, compromising professional judgement in the process. But obviously it is not as clear as that. Chris says he wishes to lose his habit.

One philosophical conception of this state of affairs offers an interesting analysis. Frankfurt[36] suggests we have 'first order' or basic desires, which might conflict with 'second order' or higher desires. Autonomy is represented by the capacity of a person rationally to repudiate a first order desire, like the usage of illicit opiates, by a second order desire, to stop. Furthermore, that capacity to rationalise our first and second order desires defines us as persons, separating us from other species who cannot. On this analysis, Chris's second order desire is becoming more powerful, and the decision to supply him with a prescription augments his autonomous one. We respect him as a person by doing so.[37]

Yet there are powerful utilitarian arguments *against* doctors prescribing drugs of addiction. A prescription may be tacitly encouraging continued use. If no doctor were permitted to prescribe in this way, doctors' experience of treating drug abusers for their addiction would be minimal. Adverse medical effects of drug use cannot be avoided, whether the drugs in question are legal, like alcohol, or illegal, like opiates. The arguments against opiate drug prescription are predominantly deontological and flow from rules and duties.

We might accept that each person has a duty to self-care, self-flourishing and survival. Given this, actions we take to use dangerous drugs conflict with this duty. Kant's ethics would support the proscription of use of addictive drugs. One formulation of his 'categorical imperative'[38] runs as follows:

> Act only according to that maxim by which you can at the same time will that it should become a universal law.[39]

In other words, it is a moral rule to do things that you would expect everyone to agree to do. It is unlikely that Chris would go along with that idea as he wishes to stop his habit, so therefore a moral rule proscribes drug use, and his GP cannot prescribe, whatever the consequences. It is worth noting that the law in England follows this maxim, up to a point:

> ... it shall not be lawful for a person –
> (a) to produce a controlled drug or
> (b) to supply or offer to supply a controlled drug to another...[40]

Kant also offered a description of human 'dignity' based on rationality. A rational being cannot be used as a means, but only as an end. On one reading, Chris wishes to use the GP as a means towards his own end of getting his drug supply. Her opinion on the best course for him is irrelevant to him. His threat violates this moral rule and thus is wrong.

None of this conceptualises Chris's addiction as an illness in the terms described above, which, by undermining his rationality offers a solution to the problem within Kantian ethics. If he is mentally 'ill', and a 'cure' in the terms with which he requests it might be a solution, it is not morally wrong. Using the Pellegrino description above, where illness is an ontological assault, addictive behaviour undermines rational, voluntary or self-determined choices. The duty of doctors is to assist in the restoration of good health and relief of suffering, in whatever the most effective way might be. If temporary prescription of opiates fulfils that duty, so be it.[41]

A contrary position would be taken by those who invest greater importance to a notion of personal responsibility. For whatever reason Chris uses harmful drugs. That in itself was an autonomous choice, and why should he not bear the consequences of that decision? At some point in the past he began his use of drugs: it might have been a first use which became a habit, it might have been the undue influence of others, it might be very difficult to establish why he did this. There may be genetic predispositions as yet ill understood.

If his GP refuses to supply methadone, temporarily or otherwise, and he is offered no other intervention, on the grounds of *desert* (which implies that Chris should simply reap the consequences of his own behaviour), that would surely be representative of a moral hardness inconsistent with the practice of medicine today. A similar principle would exclude smokers from treatment for their chronic bronchitis. But just as these smokers' illnesses are multifactorial in origin, and also due at least in part to additional factors such as living in polluted cities, it seems difficult to allocate responsibility in this way to drug addicts and exclude all treatment (*see* the case of 'Tina' in Chapter 10).

One useful view of responsibility is that it identifies what it is legitimate to punish, blame, reward or praise. Clearly if the GP simply washes her hands of Chris in this way, then she is not just blaming him, she is punishing him too.[42] That attitude is taken further by the new Drug Treatment and Testing Order that came into force in three areas of England on a pilot basis, under the Crime and Disorder Act 1998. Under this provision, drug-dependent offenders can be required to attend specialist drug treatment centres as part of the sentence of a court. It is clearly utilitarian in type and motivational in aim. Whether it is effective in reducing criminal behaviour remains to be seen.

There are now good sources of information[43] about the practical issues involved in the treatment of addicted patients, but reflection on these ethical aspects may make it easier for GPs to make the clinical decisions necessary for something which is becoming more common.

Harm to others: the ethics of intervention

The issue of doctors intervening to prevent harm to others has already been mentioned in the context of addiction. In the case of patients such as Chris, the harm is rather difficult to pin down: it consists of criminal behaviour and often cannot be attributed to a particular person. We have seen how this argument can justify continued use of addictive drugs on a 'medical prescription'. A different situation occurs when harm is more precisely definable. In the case of formal mental illness, powers are reserved by the law to prevent harm to other people when necessary. How is this justified?

> Dave has a long history of severe depression. He has been treated by his GP over some years. He has been under supervision by the community mental health team (CMHT) for about six months. He comes to the surgery one day in an agitated state, saying his wife, Elaine, has been unfaithful to him 'not for the first time'. Dave says he is going to kill her when he gets home. The GP is unable to calm Dave down and he leaves the surgery angry and distressed shouting 'You think I won't do it, don't you!'
>
> There is a waiting room full of people outside and the GP considers his next move . . .

It seems that Elaine is in danger and is at risk of harm, which might be prevented by informing the police. The GP also has a continuing duty to Dave and will doubtless keep the CMHT informed as to these events. This scenario can be conceptualised as a confidentiality issue: does he have the right to intervene by informing the police of events, with the aim of protecting Elaine? Moreover, does he have a duty to do so?

> Ought the GP to inform appropriate authorities about the danger to Dave's wife? If so, how?

In England a breach of confidentiality in a situation like this, in order to protect an identifiable person from a specific harm, is permissible under common law.[44] But there is not necessarily a duty to do so, unlike in Californian common law.[45,46] As is often the case, the law does not provide the whole answer. We need to answer the question as to the moral justification for the doctor acting, or not, as the case may be (*see* Chapter 3).

Another way of looking at it is from the point of view of *rights*. Elaine may have a *right* to the information that a dangerous husband is heading her way: this would be founded on the extent of the harm to herself, that appears to be potentially lethal.

Box 5.3 Rights theory: a reminder

- Rights are justified claims on others
- Rights impose obligations on others
- Legal rights are not necessarily moral rights
- Rights can be negative as well as positive

This sort of right is described as a negative right as it relates to non-interference. It represents a justifiable claim on the doctor for action to protect Elaine from potential harm. The GP would know that pathological jealousy could be a very dangerous situation for spouses. If he is also Elaine's GP, this claim could be said to have even greater force. As such, he would have a professional, moral and legal duty to her beyond that of an ordinary citizen. Her right as described above can only be exercised by implementing an obligation on the part of her GP to take protective action.

Another issue is whether Dave's right to behave in the way that he is doing is compromised by his mental state. If we accept that this is the case, the line of reasoning would run something like this:

- fully autonomous persons bear full rights, and obligations
- Dave lacks two components of autonomy: *understanding*,[47] by virtue of his altered mental state, secondary to his mental illness, currently under treatment. For the same reasons, he is also not *competent*[48]
- he is not fully autonomous
- he loses the right to some freedoms of action, including the right to remain at liberty[49]
- the GP is entitled to bring about that limitation of freedom by involving the police in warning Dave or Elaine.

This is not to deny Dave's right to further treatment or anything else, but it describes a justification for intervention.

A similar line of reasoning is invoked by implication when patients are compulsorily detained under the Mental Health Act 1983. For example, in Section 2, after some procedural information we see that a patient can be detained if:

> ... he ought to be so detained in the interests of his own health or safety or with a view to the protection of other persons.[50]

The Act attempts no nosological definition of 'mental illness' but allows compulsory detention, and in some sections, treatment of people with a mental disorder against their will where there is the threat of harm to others. Though it is not described in the Act, what underlies that power is the assumption of a diminished state of autonomy on the part of the patient. This is hinted at in another part of the Act where substance dependence, immorality and sexual deviancy are specifically excluded from the definition of mental illness that is given.[51]

It may be that after police intervention and psychiatric reassessment Dave is detained on these grounds: there is a threat to some other person and the use of the word 'mental illness' seems appropriate, given the known psychopathology of pathological jealousy. It is understood that the mechanics of such a detention invest the professionals with considerable powers, powers which are subject to various review procedures and safeguards. The detail of such review was brought about by the passing of the 1983 Mental Health Act over the previous 1958 Act, which allowed very little such supervision.

At the time of writing, the UK Government is considering introducing powers to detain in prison people with severe personality disorders, who may also be considered dangerous even before criminal acts have been committed.[52] Whilst this may appear draconian, in essence the psychiatrists who would be involved in the risk assessment would only be fulfilling a function similar to that of the professionals who perform assessments under the current mental health law: the quantification of risk as applied to individuals. We could ask if there is any ethical difference, even if there might be a difference in the scale of consequences.

Given these aspects it is clear that GPs need to think very carefully from an ethical perspective before invoking compulsory powers.

Harm to self: the ethics of intervention

Is a threat to the health, or life, of a patient sufficient to permit a doctor to intervene?

Francis called his GP to his house one day after telling her he had 'flu'. She checked him over and confirmed Francis' self-diagnosis. She was puzzled by the situation as Francis was not generally seen at the surgery much and the visit request 'did not fit'. It transpired, on further questioning, that Francis' wife had left him a few weeks before, with their children, and he had been sacked from his job. He was not clinically depressed or confused, but said he had no further interest in living, and had in fact taken 25 paracetamol pills the previous night, washed down with vodka in a suicide attempt. He wanted no help.

If the GP does nothing, and respects Francis' decision, he will probably die.

It could be that her *intuition* moves her to order him to hospital and set in motion compulsory powers to enforce that decision. After all, it is very difficult for a GP to sit by and watch one of her patients die: it is intuitively against a doctor's training to allow patients to die unnecessarily. Sometimes it is the easier path to press the button of intervention and know all has been done that could be done. Such an action would overrule Francis' free decision to die. But consider this:

- Francis is not depressed. There is no suggestion that a diminution of autonomy (as in Pellegrino's analysis) is present. His response to his own personal crises is to end his life and perhaps his suffering and distress. It is thought through and rational
- Francis has decided to accord less value to his life in the future than in the past. To him, life is not worth living, and should end
- the state of mind which Francis currently exhibits is not a temporary state of affairs as he has given it some considerable thought over time
- suicide is no longer illegal.[53] No one is assisting him in its commission

- refusal of treatment by a competent person is not illegal, even when 'irrational'[54] (*see* Chapter 6)
- Francis' death harms no one else. If liberty is defined as freedom not to be interfered with, his action is morally permissible. Put differently, he has a right to choose to die.

She might reflect that Francis' request for a visit undermines the first three arguments, and promotes the idea of a covert 'cry for help'. No doubt she would check this out with the patient, if she can, as well as reinforcing the likely future course. No doubt also, if she ended up accepting Francis' decision, she would keep comprehensive notes, even with a note signed by him to evidence the sequence of events. She would also get a second opinion, perhaps psychiatric, on Francis' state of mind because of the gravity of the situation. These latter actions really amount to a legal clarification of the morally driven state of affairs, however, and do not affect the moral status of Francis' decision.[55]

One further point needs consideration. On these facts, Francis is not 'mentally ill' and is allowed his autonomous choice. Some might argue that the nature of the decision implies a mental illness in itself, as if suicide can only be rationalised within the confines of a pathological mental state such as depression. Dunn[56] illustrates this line of thinking, suggesting it is inconceivable that a perfectly happy person would sit down and for no reason whatever, kill themselves. By extension such a scenario is *prima facie* evidence of mental disorder.

Clearly Francis is not perfectly happy, but neither is he ill. By contrast, Szasz[15] who denies conventional psychiatric nosology, suggests an autonomy allowing suicide should not be restricted.[57] Or as JS Mill puts it:

> the only purpose for which power can be rightfully exercised over any member of a civilised community is to prevent harm to others. His own good, either physical or moral, is not sufficient warrant[58]

In other words, the arguments that allow intervention in the case of Dave and Elaine specifically reject it in the case of Francis. These are arguments founded on the risk of harm to others, and autonomy of free agents. It matters legally because, as we shall see below, compulsion can only be invoked in the context of mental illness.

Irrational people

Francis' case could be conceptualised as one of irrationality, as already mentioned: albeit an extreme case, but nonetheless irrational. This could be taken to mean unreasoned or not sensible. Or to put it another way, behaviour taken to be irrational might be inconsistent with the qualities that are assigned to persons: the capacity for evaluative, descriptive or analytical thought. Since we do not find, broadly speaking, such qualities in other species, they are innately human and therefore define at least one of the attributes of people.

Irrational behaviour seems to go against this. Sometimes this can be conceptualised as 'illness' deserving of a doctor's care and the mental illness problems described above fall into this category. It is evident in severe psychotic illness, where fragmentation of thought is a feature, that irrational behaviour can follow a 'pathological' mental state. The same description would hold for a toxic confusional state.

But where a patient holds views, or behaves in a way that is irrational in the above sense – where such attributes are unreasoned – is that a state requiring medical intervention? A discussion of this problem must apply only to mature adults, for the obvious reason that children have not yet realised their full potential for the attributes described, though such a potential is evolving, and is not an all or nothing phenomenon (*see* Chapter 8).[59]

A patient returned this note to a GP's practice, written across the top of a cervical smear invitation.

'NOT INTERESTED SEEN TOO MANY RELATIVES, FRIENDS, DIE OF THE CURE, IF I DEVELOP CANCER, I'LL DIE OF IT. NEVER WILL I EXCEPT TREATMENT FOR CANCER, FOR MYSELF. BESIDES THE SO-CALLED TESTS ARE FLAWED'
(sic)

As has been seen in Chapter 4, such tests may indeed be flawed, so this observation may not in itself be irrational. Leaving that aside, does this 'advance statement' indicate that it is unreasoned?

What ought a GP or the practice nurse to do on its receipt?

In contrast, consider a patient who is advised to have an endoscopy to investigate late onset dyspepsia, refuses it and steadfastly holds to this view, despite explanation, because of fear of the procedure. Phobic anxiety of this type is unreasoned but real for the person involved. Should the doctor accept this as a freely autonomous decision or nag her into submission in her best interests?

It is not easy for a doctor to accept a patient's decision that is not obviously in that patient's best interests, if best interests is defined only in medical terms such as prolongation or improved quality of life. But if irrationality is acknowledged as a human quality akin to a religious belief, for example, then it seems easier to respect such a decision.

Conclusion

In matters which concern mental health, current discussion, morally speaking, is focused on the limits of paternalism as translated into law. The issue of compulsion is particularly relevant as the grounds for compulsory treatment are under review. From the GP's perspective this has the potential to make lawful compulsory community treatment, which will break the link between detention and treatment. If this happens, GPs will be more involved with compulsion, and need to reflect more on its moral justification. To do this it is necessary to explore the notion of consent in more detail, and this follows in the next chapter.

At a more practical level, ethical examination of some of the common clinical problems in mental illness has not shown that they should be considered any differently from common physical ones. It lends support to the oft-quoted maxim that GPs should always think of patients and their problems in physical, social and psychological terms.

References and notes

1   Lurie A (1967) *Imaginary Friends*. Abacus, London.
2   The standard secondary care textbook of mental illness ethics is Chodoff P and Bloch S (eds) (1991) *Psychiatric Ethics*. Oxford Medical, Oxford.

3   Scull AT (1979) *Museums of Madness*. Allen Lane, London.

4   Wright AF (1996) Unrecognised psychiatric illness in general practice. *Br J Gen Pract*. **46**(407): 327–8. This article highlights the difference between GPs and academic researchers in making psychiatric diagnoses in general practice.

5   Jenkins KR, Jenkins R and Mann A (1996) Long term outcome of patients with neurotic illness in general practice. *BMJ*. **313**: 26–8.

6   McWhinney I (1996) The importance of being different. *Br J Gen Pract*. **46**: 433–6. (William Pickles Lecture RCGP 1996.)

7   Recent correspondence in the *BMJ* has focused on new definitions for general practice. *See* Heath I, Evans P and van Weel C (2000) The specialist of the discipline of general practice. *BMJ*. **320**: 326–7 and discussion in various authors (2000). *BMJ*. **321**: 173–4.

8   This assumes that GPs and other healthcare professionals can and should promote health as well as deal with perceived illness. Health could be defined as a sense of well-being, a positive notion necessary to pursue other personal goals. *See* Downie RS and Calman KC (1994) *Healthy Respect* (2e). Oxford University Press, Oxford, pp. 87–90.

9   Neighbour R (1997) *The Inner Consultation*. Petroc Press, Newbury, pp. 35–6.

10 McWhinney describes this as an 'organismic rather than mechanistic metaphor of biology'. *See* note 6.

11 Craig TKJ and Brown GW (1994) Goal frustration and life events in the aetiology of painful gastrointestinal disorder. In: P Steptoe and D Wardle (eds) *Psychosocial Processes and Health: a reader*. Cambridge University Press, Edinburgh.

12 A full account of this problem can be found in Clare A (1979) The disease concept in psychiatry. In: P Hill, R Murray and A Thorley (eds) *Essentials of Postgraduate Psychiatry*. Academic Press, London.

13 American Psychiatric Association (1994) *Diagnostic and Statistical Manual of Mental Disorders* (4e) (DSM 1V). This is an example of categorised description of mental health.

14 Richard Asher reminds us that one illness is the same as another if it is indistinguishable from it. *See* British Medical Association (1994) *Talking Sense or A Sense of Asher*. BMA, London.

15 Szasz T (1992) *The Myth of Mental Illness*. Paladin, London and Boyers P and Orvill R (eds) (1993) *Laing and the Anti-psychiatrists*. Penguin, Harmondsworth offer a good review of this area.

16 Butler CC, Evans M *et al*. (1999) The heartsink patient revisited. *Br J Gen Pract*. **49**: 230–3.

17 Salmon P, Peters S and Stanley I (1999) Patients perceptions of medical explanations for somatization disorders: qualitative analysis. *BMJ*. **318**: 372–5.

18 O'Carroll A (1995) Heartsink Patients. *Rheumatol Pract.* **Sept.** He criticises a conception of illness as 'good' if identifiable pathologically, and 'bad' if vague, woolly and unverifiable.

19 Konrad M (1983) A defence of medical paternalism: maximising patients' autonomy. *J Med Ethics.* **9**: 38–44.

20 Pellegrino ED (1979) Toward a reconstruction of medical morality. *J Med Philosophy.* **4**(4): 32–56.

21 O'Neill O (1984) Paternalism and partial autonomy. *J Med Ethics* (original emphasis). **10**: 173–8.

22 Toon P (1999) *Toward a philosophy of general practice: a study of the virtuous practitioner.* RCGP, London. Occasional Paper 78, Ch. 7.

23 Mill JS (1990) A crisis in my mental history. In: *Autobiography,* Ch. 5 or in Glover J (ed.) *Utilitarianism and its Critics.* Macmillan for a short description of how philosophers can get depressed.

24 Middleton H and Shaw I (2000) Distinguishing mental illness in primary care. *BMJ.* **320**: 1420–1.

25 These are validated instruments for the assessment of mental illnesses, born originally of academic research, but useful in clinical practice.

26 Ashton J (1980) *Everyday Psychiatry.* Update Books, London, Ch. 1.

27 Denig P and Bradley C suggest that the intensity of drug marketing sponsors an atmosphere where all ills just need the right pill. Denig P and Bradley C (1998) *Prescribing in Primary Care.* Oxford University Press, Oxford, Ch. 5.

28 Neighbour's 'political model' of illness. *See* note 9.

29 Kendrick T (1996) Prescribing anti-depressants in general practice. *BMJ.* **313**: 829–30. We are reminded that research suggests antidepressants are useful only in 'major depression', i.e. low mood or loss of interest or pleasure for two weeks **and** four of the following symptoms present: appetite change, sleep disorder, fatigue/anergia, poor concentration, guilt, retardation or suicidal thoughts. In minor depression 'don't just do something, sit there', referring to the drug prescription issue only, we suspect. However, does evidence of efficacy define beneficence?

30 This whole area is developed in more detail by Higgs R (1999) Depression in general practice. In: C Dowrick and L Frith (eds) *General Practice and Ethics: uncertainty and responsibility.* Routledge, London.

31 Marmot M and Brunner E (1991) Alcohol and cardiovascular disease: the status of the U-shaped curve. *BMJ.* **303**: 565–8.

32 Doll R, Peto R, Hall E *et al.* (1994) Mortality in relation to consumption of alcohol: 13 years observation on male British doctors. *BMJ.* **309**: 911–98.

33 General Medical Council (1997) *Serious Communicable Diseases.* GMC, London, para 2. Also General Medical Council (1997) *Good Medical Practice.* GMC, London.

34 Hindler C, King M, Nazareth I *et al.* (1996) Characteristics of drug misusers and their perceptions of general practitioner care. *Br J Gen Pract.* **46**: 149–52.

35 Keen J, Rowse G, Mathers N *et al.* (2000) Can methadone maintenance for heroin dependent patients retained in general practice reduce criminal conviction rates and time spent in prison? *Br J Gen Pract.* **50**: 48–9.

36 Frankfurt HG (1971) Freedom of the will and the concept of a person. *J Philosophy.* **68**: 5–20.

37 The clinical counterpart of this model from philosophy can be found in Whitehead B (1997) Counselling drug users. In: B Beaumont (ed.) *Care of Drug Users in General Practice – a harm minimisation approach.* Radcliffe Medical Press, Oxford.

38 For Kant, these are rules that must be obeyed.

39 Kant I (1785) *Groundwork of Metaphysics of Morals.*

40 Misuse of Drugs Act 1971, para. 4 [1].

41 Efficacy is a loaded term. In the biomedical model, it approximates to success in outcome, preferably from an evidence base. It is implicitly utilitarian.

42 Glover J (1970) *Responsibility.* Routledge, London.

43 DoH (1999) *Drug Misuse and Dependence – guidelines on clinical management.* HMSO, London.

44 W v Egdell (1990) 1 *All ER:* 835.

45 Tarasoff v Regents of University of California (1976) **131** *Cal Rptr:* 14 (*Cal Sup Ct*).

46 Applebaum PS (1985) in the *American Journal of Psychiatry* **142**: 425–9 refers to lack of specific legislation in the UK as to informing those at risk of threat of violence generally.

47 Understanding in this context implies knowledge and its application. That knowledge includes a moral aspect, which if Dave was not 'ill', he would not lack.

48 Defined in phenomenological terms.

49 An interesting further discussion of this point is found in Dworkin R (1977) *Taking Rights Seriously,* Duckworth, New York, Ch. 12.

50 Mental Health Act 1983. Part II s2 (1) b.

51 Mental Health Act 1983 Part I s1 (2) and (3).

52 HM Government (1999) *Reform of the Mental Health Act 1983: proposals for consultation.* The Stationery Office, London, Annex 3.

53 Suicide Act 1961 s1.

54 *See* Hewson B (1999) The law on managing patients who deliberately harm themselves and refuse treatment. *BMJ.* **319**: 905–7 for a full legal analysis.

55 An accessible philosophical account of suicide is to be found in Glover J (1990) *Causing Death and Saving Lives.* Penguin, Harmondsworth, Ch. 13.

56 Dunn C (1998) *Ethical Issues in Mental Illness.* Ashgate, Aldershot, p. 15 *et seq.*
57 David Hume (1794) Of suicide. In: P Singer (ed.) *Applied Ethics.* Oxford University Press, Oxford.
58 Mill JS (1985) *3 Essays: on liberty, representative government, and the subjection of women.* 1859 reprinted 1975. Oxford University Press, Oxford.
59 The law recognises this fact.

CHAPTER SIX

The elements of consent: information and understanding

Summary

This area of clinical practice can cause an unwarranted degree of confusion. Yet assessment of competence for consent to treatment is a task with which GPs must be involved: guidance as to the ethical and legal issues will assist the process.

- Forms of consent
- Competence and capacity
- The influence of others
- Understanding and risk
- Proxies
- Constraints on consent.

... I suffer therefore I am, and so in perfect freedom can tell the doctor what I think of him and the wild ideas he pulls out after he has collaborated in cutting open my stomach for nothing, errare humanum est, *I say to him ...*[1]

Forms of consent

It seems almost obvious to describe consent by a person to a procedure or other clinical intervention as their agreement to it. That it is not so obvious is evidenced by the fact that, in a medical context, doctors do things that otherwise would be regarded rather strangely; most people do not, for example, ask potentially intrusive questions of others, or insert tubing into other people's orifices. What demands a form of consent in all these clinical situations is the nature of a doctor's activity and the special relationship between doctor and patient.

GPs are given permission by virtue of their special position as doctors to behave in this way and thus require consent from the patient to do so. That consent might take several forms.

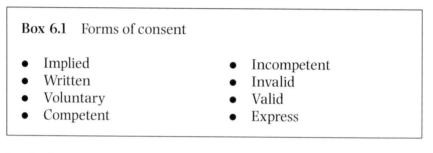

Box 6.1 Forms of consent

- Implied
- Written
- Voluntary
- Competent
- Incompetent
- Invalid
- Valid
- Express

Implied consent could be thought of as a rather tenuous notion. What is suggested is that the actions or words of the patient imply agreement to a particular action, even if not made clear, or express. One could say that when someone sits down and presents their arm in the appropriate way after discussion, then consent to venepuncture is present, even if the GP or practice nurse has not actually said: 'May I take your blood now please?'

In a very old case from New York, an emigrant to the USA challenged this idea after she had been vaccinated for smallpox in a long line of other emigrants, arms proffered, on the docks in 1891. She lost her case, as the court held she had implied consent by her acceptance of the vaccination at the time.[2]

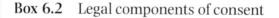

Box 6.2 Legal components of consent

- Intention
- Voluntariness
- Competence

Box 6.2 shows the legally required aspects of a valid consent by a patient. If any of these three aspects is in doubt, then the consent is invalid. That might have implications for the doctor, but it is still necessary to ask why this might be ethically unsound. Compare this list with Box 6.3 detailing the components of autonomy as described by Beauchamp and Childress.[3]

Box 6.3   Components of autonomy

Understanding
Freedom from controlling influences
Capacity

As one might expect, these two lists are rather similar; law flows from ethics, and not vice versa, as has been said repeatedly. Let us deal in a little more detail with these aspects.

Competence and capacity

Readers will note that the terms *competence* and *capacity* are frequently used in medical, philosophical and legal writing. Doctors should regard them as essentially synonymous. What is being described is the *ability* of people to make decisions; but specific to medical ethics is an ability to make decisions about *diagnosis* and *treatment*. Sometimes it requires little analysis to reach the conclusion that no capacity exists in a patient. Babies most clearly represent this. In this case, decisions must fall to a proxy, and the most obvious proxy for a baby is a parent. A baby has no capacity for rational or evaluative thought at this stage in his development and this seems to underlie his incompetent status.

This is not to say that decisions about treatment or anything else are always rational, in the sense of health preservation or logic, or that doctors are required to accept them when they are not. A string of cases at law, where people who hold that transfusions of blood are immoral and impermissible, has shown this. Jehovah's Witnesses are people with such views, preferring not to receive such a treatment even when life may be at risk.[4] What underlies the acceptance of this at law is the principle that people can make life-threatening decisions for themselves as long as the other components of valid consent are applied, and the religious beliefs that inform them are 'core values'. Therefore, a personal moral rule based on a religious value is determinative. This will allow non-transfusion of a Jehovah's Witness *in extremis* whose life would otherwise be saved. His 'best interests' are not necessarily served by the saving of his life. Clearly this view challenges the rational view of the world that most doctors would claim to espouse.

Gordon was a severely affected schizophrenic patient. He was in hospital under a long-term section of the Mental Health Act and was improving. Discharge to a community residential home was envisaged fairly soon. Unfortunately, Gordon developed a subacute bowel obstruction and had to be admitted to the general hospital. Needing surgery for this problem, his surgeon was not able to gain his consent. His psychiatrist could not persuade him either. The risk of death if he was not operated on was substantial, rated by the surgeon at 50%. The hospital doctors called in Gordon's GP to the hospital to assess him and to try to persuade him to accept the operation. In conversation his GP found that Gordon fully understood the situation.

Some GPs when confronted with a story like this might say that Gordon is not competent by virtue of his psychiatric illness and thus can be forced into surgery in his own interests. They might also say that this defines the difference with a Jehovah's Witness decision. Gordon is functioning mentally at a lower level, reduced by virtue of his schizophrenic illness and implying a reduced capacity. This would be a superficial view, however, because it takes no account of Gordon's *actual* understanding and decision making. He may be psychotic, which influences his view, of reality, but that does not necessarily undermine his capacity for evaluative thought in other areas.

The ethical principle here is that patients ought to be allowed to make their own decisions, whatever the outcome, to a degree commensurate with their capacity. That capacity may be altered, but is only absent in certain situations, such as in the baby mentioned above. Even though Gordon's freedom is constrained by being under section, he still has the freedom to determine some of his actions. This is a deontological precept. Respect for persons, founded on individual value, underlies it. Were it to be a determinative utilitarian principle based on outcome Gordon would have surgery against his wishes.

English law upholds the deontological principle, and would not, given certain factors, oblige a patient like Gordon to have surgery, much as the doctors might wish it. The Code of Practice issued with the Mental Health Act 1983 states that for an individual to have capacity, he must understand the nature, purpose and likely effects of the proposed medical treatment, in other words:

- understand in broad terms the nature of the treatment
- understand its principal benefits and risks
- understand what will be the consequences of not receiving the proposed treatment
- possess the capacity to make a choice.

It must be remembered that:

- any assessment as to an individual's capacity has to be made in relation to a particular proposal
- capacity in an individual with a mental disorder can be variable over time
- all assessments of an individual's capacity should be fully recorded in the patient's medical notes.[5]

In the case of *Re C*, very similar to Gordon in this hypothetical case, three criteria were held to define capacity to consent.[6] The patient must be able to:

- comprehend and retain treatment information
- believe the information
- weigh it in the balance to arrive at a choice.

This is obviously more than a simple understanding of the problem.[7] It might be that Gordon therefore does have capacity to make real consent or otherwise to his operation, whatever the outcome. That is not the case for his mental illness, where the issue of capacity might actually be sidelined. He is in hospital on a long-term compulsory order. Almost by definition any capacity he might have to determine his own future with respect to his mental illness and treatment has been overridden.

In this story we do not know why this is so, but if Gordon has capacity to determine his own fate with regard to his abdominal problem, why is this not so with regard to his psychiatric state? The obvious answer is a possible risk to others, as in the case of Dave, above. However, a powerful argument has been advanced by MIND and others that the *Re C* principles should be applied to mental illness as well.[8] If this was the case, Gordon's detention and treatment for his schizophrenia could only be lawful on a capacity basis, rather than as a presumed risk to others.

This approach has the conceptual benefit for doctors of blending illness models in the way described above, such that they think ethically and legally similarly about mental and physical illness. It is not consonant with the current proposals for a change in UK mental health law.

Special considerations arise in the case of children that are dealt with in Chapter 8. For the purpose of this chapter it is notable that a conception of *assent* has grown in childcare, where value is attached to a child's agreement prior to treatment rather than a reliance on consent on his behalf by an adult.

The influence of others

The ethical principle of autonomy, according to Beauchamp and Childress, requires the moral agent to be free of controlling influences akin to the legal principle of voluntariness. There is a vast and complex philosophical literature on free will, in which positions are taken between those who deny freedom of will exists at all (*determinists*) and those who argue that we have complete freedom to act (*libertarians*). Control, in this context, seems to be a strong version of influence, both of which may affect decisions inappropriately. Another description might be coercion.

Hurwitz recounts a striking example of coercion by a GP that ultimately worked to the benefit of patient and family. An elderly lady was tying up more and more community services as she steadfastly refused, in clear consciousness, admission to hospital for treatment of a treatable skin tumour. The arrival of a new GP on the scene who brooked no such refusal broke the impasse in a deteriorating situation and facilitated her removal to secondary care, against her immediate wishes. She recovered.[9]

Morally speaking, the GP in the case acted from a consequentialist perspective, and was justified by the outcome. Alternatively, this sort of case could be conceptualised as justified paternalism, though it must be recognised that it exemplifies a non-autonomous decision on the part of the patient. Autonomy was outweighed by beneficence, where beneficence is defined in biomedical terms.

More extreme cases arise under 1993 statute law in the USA where patients with tuberculosis (TB) can be treated compulsorily to prevent spread of multiresistant disease. It is clearly an example of non-consensual treatment where, within a state programme of TB control, some very uncooperative people can be detained against their will to facilitate a cure. What seems to be a justification for this sort of paternalism is the fact that multiresistant TB is a disease of disadvantaged people like the homeless or the poor, so that measures such as this combat any apparent 'silent fatalism'. The influence of others, in this case the state via statute, is rarely more obvious.[10,11]

Harriet is 85 years old and lives alone. She has severe osteoarthrosis and has problems transferring between her bed, chair and commode. Her care manager supervises Harriet's twice daily visits by the home care team and is very concerned at the risk of falls leading to serious injury. She asks Harriet's GP to visit with a view to admitting her to a nursing home as the whole care package seems to be breaking down.

Although rather deaf, Harriet makes her opposition to this plan clear to the GP, volubly and rationally. The care manager does not accept this, citing the risks not only to Harriet, but also to her staff from back injuries from the strain of lifting her about. After some weeks of this, Harriet gives way and agrees to enter a nursing home for further care.

This is an increasingly familiar scenario as our population ages; more and more people are becoming dependent on professional or family carers. GPs often find themselves caught between the professional and the patient, as they try to work out the best course.

Were the professionals right to persuade Harriet to leave her home?

The question to answer here is whether Harriet did make an autonomous decision, or whether it was constrained by the influence of the professionals. Harriet is competent, it seems, and one must ask why this would not be enough to allow her to bear the risk of injury by remaining at home. A utilitarian might say that the potential outcome carried greater weight than her freely held autonomous decision, and if this is right, both professionals took a utilitarian position in coercing her into admission. They may have concerns of criticism in the event of a coroner's inquest should Harriet die of a 'preventable' injury. However, in summary we might describe this professional opinion as beneficence outweighing autonomy.

Conversely, it is a powerful argument that would allow Harriet to stay in her own home, in full possession of the facts, even at risk to herself. There seems little harm to others by her remaining there save the carers' backs (which is probably preventable), so what we have is an example of a negative conception of liberty. The professionals exercised a degree of persuasion or coercion to bring about Harriet's eventual grudging acceptance of her transfer, thereby removing one of the conditions of a free autonomous choice.

Occasionally, statutory powers can be used to overwhelm the will of old people living in severely insanitary conditions, and unable to care for themselves, and have them removed to an appropriate place – usually a hospital or other care facility. This legal device, under the National Assistance Act 1948 (s47), is for competent persons in this situation and only undertaken in rare cases: about 250 per year in the UK. Such persons are often referred to as demonstrating the 'Diogenes syndrome'.[12] Mental health law is not relevant to this sort of case as there is no mental illness: the resistance of an old person to cooperate with health or social care professionals does not fit into any nosological variety of mental illness.

More subtle kinds of external influence may arise from the family of a patient. Indeed, it would be surprising if the people that we love and live with did not have an influence on our decision; it is after all a kind of teamwork we indulge in with our closest friends and family. Where influence may be 'undue' was examined in a 1993 case in England. *Re T* had many important issues to examine but of interest here is the role of others in manipulating a patient's decision. T was pregnant and involved in a car crash. She was not a Jehovah's Witness, but soon after arrival at hospital she had a conversation with her mother who was. After this T announced that she would not have a transfusion of blood should it become necessary.[13]

We should remember that common law in England would:

1   allow a competent refusal of treatment, including transfusion, even unto death, and
2   not allow another person, even a mother, to consent or refuse on behalf of another.

However in this case, that refusal only became apparent after T's mother had a private conversation with her. In the event the hospital doctors deemed a transfusion necessary and a High Court judge sanctioned it in T's best interests. He considered that undue pressure had been put on T such that her refusal was not valid: it had been corrupted, or in legal terms 'vitiated'.

At appeal, the three judges each made contributions that illuminated the more general aspects of 'undue influence'. Lord Donaldson described it thus:

> when considering the effect of outside influences, two aspects can be of crucial importance. First the strength of will of the patient. One who is very tired, in pain or depressed will be much less able to resist having his will overborne than one who is rested, free from pain or cheerful. Second, the relationship of the persuader to the patient may be of crucial importance. The influence of parents on their children or of one spouse on another can be, but is by no means necessarily, much stronger than would be the case in other relationships. Persuasion based on religious beliefs can be much more compelling and the fact that arguments based on religious beliefs are being deployed by someone in a very close relationship with the patient will give them added force and should alert the doctors to the possibility – no more – that the patient's capacity or will to decide has been overborne. In other words, the patient may not mean what he says.

Judge Butler-Sloss said more succinctly that:

> it has long been recognised that an influence can be subtle, insidious, pervasive, and where religious beliefs are involved, especially powerful. It may also be powerful between close relatives where one may be in a dominant position vis-à-vis the other.

As this is a legal case, the judges are all examining T's situation from the point of view of voluntariness. Was her refusal of a blood transfusion really voluntary or did it spring from the undue influence of her mother? There were other aspects to the case based on T's competence, but our interest here is to work back from the law and focus on the aspects that come to light that would undermine an autonomous decision by reducing freedom from controlling influence, analogous to legal voluntariness. Their lordships describe reduced strength of will, the role of illness or pain, religious beliefs, and close relationships as all being factors doctors should be cautious about when assessing whether decisions are free and uncoerced. It is difficult to put it better than they did.

Understanding and risk

For a patient's decision to be freely autonomous, it must be replete with understanding. It is necessary to clarify what this might mean.

The original meaning of the word 'doctor' is that of a *teacher*, so it could be said that GPs should assume the historical role and enhance patients' understanding of their situations. Doctors are in a better position to fulfil this having maximised their own understanding of the patient's problems; this is best done by listening to the patient.[14] In recent years, the vast literature on consultation skills, particularly familiar to GPs in training, bears witness to this.

Freeling and Gask summarised it thus: some patients want to know more than they are told, and some do not, having 'absolute, uncritical confidence in their doctor's skills'. They see this as a balance between paternalism and autonomy requiring, in itself, specific skills, and they offer a clinical framework for so doing.[15] Several areas spring to mind as the things a patient might need to know before deciding anything – effects, consequences, risks, burdens, benefits, side-effects: the list could be endless. We need to consider the question:

> What is the 'right' amount of information to put across?

Merely transmitting information would not seem to be sufficient, as this does not necessarily include understanding. But to commit professionals to ensuring complete understanding of all aspects of a decision that a patient has to face would be onerous in the extreme, and it might not always be possible.

Purposefully telling untruths, even if they seem to be 'better' for the patient at the time, is a course of action that these days would be difficult to justify. Higgs, in a review of the whole subject, ended up unconvinced by any arguments for lying to patients, and made the point that this was ultimately corrosive of the doctor–patient relationship.[16] It must also be recognised that there are some patients who will have no understanding, or at least diminished understanding, of their options and thus will have only a partial autonomy to bring to bear on a clinical decision: the example of the baby is obvious. Less obvious are patients with learning difficulties in whom a *full* understanding might be impossible to achieve. That is not to say that they should not be offered a chance to understand to the maximum possible, and participate in decision making accordingly.

However, a recent review suggested current healthcare practice in the UK did not serve adults with learning difficulties well in the area of decision making, citing *inter alia* over-reliance on proxies, and organisational and attitudinal barriers.[17] In practical terms we may have some way to go in this area.

Most of the English law on the issue of information, and what is the proper information to divulge to the patient, has arisen from disputes in the aftermath of surgical mishaps. These cases are medical negligence cases where the accusation of the claimant is generally that an appropriate degree of risk information was not communicated, and this constitutes a ground for an action. It is useful to be aware of the principles that are examined because they apply to non-surgical situations as well, and by extension, any medical treatment, right down to an everyday prescription issue.

The notion of 'informed consent' is crucial here. Procedures are lawful if the patient is adequately informed to make a proper consent. In England, broadly speaking that depends on the doctor's view (though this is slowly changing) but in the USA it depends on the patient's view. Lest this may seem rather an oblique statement, let us examine it in more detail.

Until a few years ago English law relied on what is known as the *Bolam* test to judge the standard of information given to a patient.[18] This standard is based upon that which a doctor, following the responsible practice of his colleagues, would reasonably divulge. In America, common law evolved differently, to come to what is known as the 'reasonable patient' test, i.e. what a reasonable patient might expect to want to know. That said, in latter years, English courts have begun to want to examine the practices of doctors more objectively, rather than accept the practice because it complies with that of a body of doctors. Following the case of *Bolitho*, English courts expect the responsible practice to 'withstand logical analysis'.[19] Given a doctor's training, it does not seem unreasonable that this is so. How might this apply to Ingrid?

Ingrid was 38 years old and had three children. She used oral contraception and had done since the birth of her youngest child 2 years previously. She felt her family was now complete and wanted to stop using a hormone-based family planning method. She talked to a practice nurse about this and considered her options, finally deciding on a coil, which was fitted one afternoon by her GP. All was well at her follow-up at 6 weeks, but about a year later she missed a period and found out she was pregnant a few weeks later on. Ingrid was very distressed about this and would not consider termination of the pregnancy on religious grounds. She said she would never have stopped the combined pill had she known about the chances of pregnancy. The GP removed the coil. Ingrid delivered a healthy child 7 months later.

It seems she did not appreciate the failure rate of the intrauterine contraceptive device (IUCD), or at least that is her interpretation of the information given to her by her advisers beforehand. According to the *Bolam* test, if it is the practice of a responsible body of GPs not to give this information, then it is lawful in England, if the courts agree that that practice is reasonable.

In the USA, the courts would ask the question: 'Would a reasonable patient want to know the failure rate of this IUCD?' to which the answer would no doubt be 'Yes' and the action of not informing Ingrid would be unlawful as her consent was vitiated thereby (*see* note 13). This latter requirement has become known as the doctrine of informed consent, although obviously either American or British practice could be described as such. These legal observations help us only to the extent of determining lawfulness; they do not argue for the *ethical* requirement to ensure that Ingrid *understood* the full implications of the coil as a contraceptive and its failure rate. She had the *right* to know. She was facing a problem in understanding the failure rate of coils *versus* oral contraception. It can be difficult to explain statistical functions such as pregnancies per woman year, or other contraception performance indicators. There is evidence that we do not do it very well despite our best efforts, but also that we need to do it differently for different people.[20] Whether Ingrid's nurse and doctor achieved this is open to question, but if understanding is a precondition of an *autonomous* decision, it seems unlikely that they did.

A degree of understanding, in this context, is perhaps best expressed as a process of 'shared decision making', requiring as Tate puts it:

> enough time to allow a sufficient exchange of information ... a bespoke message based on medical knowledge, ideas, concerns, expectations, effects and feelings of both parties engaged in this communication.[21]

It is a formidable task to embrace all of these in every consultation decision in general practice. In reality, short cuts are taken because of the pressure of time. We must acknowledge that, on this analysis of information and understanding, such short cuts have a dubious ethical basis.

Something of the nature of risk has already been examined in Chapter 4. It is clear that part of the problem about risk is that people have conceptual difficulties with its understanding, which in turn can degrade the quality of autonomy inherent in a risk-related decision like that of Ingrid. The derivation of the word is actually from an old Portuguese word meaning 'to dare' and this does not sit easily with a reasoned approach to clinical decisions.

Many writers have alluded to the problems in achieving understanding by quoting figures at patients: risks of complications being $x\%$ or y in 100 000 cases per year or many other variations on a theme.[22,23] A more detailed approach to achieving an understanding of risk, and by extension, a greater degree of autonomy, is suggested by Calman and Royston, who talk of risk 'dialects' to enhance such understanding.[24] Given an intrinsic difficulty with numerical data, which risk assessments inevitably propound, they suggest that a common 'language' might be logarithmic. The 'dialects' of this language are formed by new means of presentation: visual, analogous or verbal. For example, the risk of death due to oral contraception each year could be explained as follows:

> On the best evidence currently available, the chance of someone being affected by this hazard is 1 in 1 000 000. This is magnitude 7 on a risk scale. This level of risk is analogous to the chance of an individual being selected at random out of a line of people standing one metre apart stretching from Land's End to John O'Groats. You could expect to find one person affected in every large city or county of Great Britain. Many people would judge this risk to be minimal or negligible compared to the risks of normal living.[24,25]

It is not difficult to see that enhancement of risk understanding for our patients can be dramatically improved by this or other such means. This is becoming increasingly relevant in areas such as measures towards prevention of ischaemic heart disease, where risks are multifactorial in origin as mentioned already in Chapter 4.[26]

A male smoker of 60 years with borderline lipids and blood pressure has an absolute risk of a cardiac event of 30%. Given his full understanding of his risk, and refusal to stop smoking, should he be given a statin to reduce the chances of a myocardial infarction?

Proxies

Some mention has already been made of the role of proxy decision-makers. These are people who take decisions for others, where circumstances may seem to require it. Chapter 8 deals with this problem with respect to children, but there is the issue of proxy decisions in adults. What then might be the justification for one competent adult to decide for another?

The situation is only going to arise where there is diminished autonomy, by virtue of any of the three components discussed above, and a decision needs to be made on behalf of the patient.

Jack was 35 and suffered from moderate learning difficulties, attending an adult training centre five days a week. Kelly, his friend at the centre of some years standing, had similar difficulties and epilepsy too.

Both were registered with a local GP who came in to do a session each week there. By chance, while she was doing her weekly session at the centre, Jack slipped and injured his arm. He was taken to casualty where a fracture was found. The trauma registrar phoned and asked the GP to sign her consent form for reduction of the fracture, as Jack self-evidently could not. While she was mulling this over, Kelly started a fit and did not stop after 5 minutes. The doctor administered rectal diazepam and Kelly slowly recovered.

This rather eventful morning illustrates a number of the principles at issue here.

In treating Kelly, the GP is working without consent: there is no understanding on the patient's part, not only because of her pre-existent mental state (which we assume to be of that degree) but also because she is unconscious and fitting. The GP administers the treatment under the principle of beneficence, since to do otherwise would be maleficent. It is a quite straightforward ethical underpinning of treatment.

The legal implications of the GP's action are more complex. Whether Kelly has learning difficulties or not, no one can consent for her, in law. The lawfulness of the treatment for her fits is founded on the principle of *necessity*. A judge in one of the leading cases in this area suggested that the emergency nature of certain interventions drives the necessity principle, and this is the case in the GP's treatment of Kelly. Delay is not reasonable. Had a treatment to stop her fits not been administered, harm and possibly death might have ensued. But the treatment, it is clear, is outside of any consent.[27] The GP in this kind of situation has been described as a 'quasi-proxy', a person empowered under law to carry out a treatment.[28]

The trauma registrar is asking considerably more than that in his phone call to the GP: he is asking her to be a proxy *per se* for what seems to be a necessary treatment. The legal base to this is also quite complex and interesting. Prior to the Mental Health Act 1959, the Crown and courts had an ancient power of *prerogative* to consent for mentally disordered persons, or in the phraseology of the time 'lunatics, idiots and others of unsound mind'. This was known as the *parens patriae* jurisdiction, and dates back to the sixteenth century. It lapsed with the introduction of statute law in the 1959 Act (*see* Chapter 8).[29] In essence there is no general power of consent by the state for medical treatment, or anything else, unless statutory procedures are followed. Even the guardianship powers of the 1983 Mental Health Act do not allow for consent to medical treatment.[30]

So how is the trauma registrar to proceed? No doubt he is grasping for some appropriate procedure to follow, but he has not happened on the right one. His GP cannot consent for Jack, even if she knows him well, and would be well advised to decline the offer. She might make a statement in his hospital notes declaring the fracture setting to be in Jack's best interests, referencing her previous knowledge of him, but this cannot be considered in any sense a consent. The trauma registrar becomes a 'quasi-proxy' and has to proceed without consent in Jack's best interests, and of necessity, under common law.

It is obvious in Jack's case that his best interests are served by the setting of his arm, but we are reminded by the GMC that this is not always so. They set out the considerations needed when defining best interests in persons without competence.

- Options for treatment or investigation which are clinically indicated.
- Any evidence of the patient's previously expressed preferences, including advance statements.
- Knowledge of the patient's background, e.g. culture, religion, employment.
- Patient's preferences given by a third party: family, carer, parent.
- Which option least restricts the patient's future choices, where there are several reasonable options.[31]

Several further points arise from the GMC summary above.

First, the role of relatives in the care and decision making of incompetent patients is being debated at the time of writing, and it is likely that a new statutory framework will ensue in a review of the Mental Health Act. There has been much academic writing as well as formal government consultation in this important area.[32] Roles of relatives will probably enlarge and this will have an impact on the sort of situations described above.

Second, the GMC describes a different view of autonomy in the fifth consideration given above. It is easy to imagine the principle of autonomy rather simplistically as a conception of free choice, with philosophers arguing about how 'free' is 'free'. What the GMC hint at is rather what autonomy might be for, that is to say, the capacity to exert further free choices in the future. It is as if the person with learning difficulties, being deprived of some choices by virtue of his condition, should therefore look to his doctors to maximise his future choices in the selection of treatments. This might be described as 'fostering' autonomy.

Third, reference is made to the importance of culture and background in assessing options for treatment. This has other implications as we shall see below.

Constraints on consent

Ethics has a capacity to confuse, perhaps because clear and concise ethical answers to problems are elusive. Nowhere is this more evident than in the discussion of *relativism* or in the notion that one person's interpretation of ethics is right and another's is wrong. Arguments can arise when we consider whether or not consent is possible.

So far in this chapter the overarching theme is that autonomy as a principle 'trumps' other principles, so that the role of doctors is to give effect wherever possible to decisions by patients that are self-made, even if the decisions seem irrational. What might happen if such decisions conflict with other people's moral rules, or laws, and how is the problem resolved?

Leo was 12 years old and the subject of a child protection enquiry. It seemed that his father had beaten him with a cane after he had misbehaved one day. He had stolen some money from a shop. It came to light because a neighbour had heard shrieks from their house one afternoon.

His GP was invited to a case conference in due course, as was the health visitor of the practice. They knew of no previous child protection issues relevant to the case. Leo was otherwise well parented. After taking views from those present, the chairperson concluded at the end of the conference that this was a case of over-chastisement and took no further action, other than a warning.

Presumably Leo did not consent to his corporal punishment in the aftermath of his errant behaviour. As a proxy, was his father entitled to commit the act? He would likely as not argue that this was actually in Leo's best interests as a deterrent for the future, and that it reinforced a moral rule with which we should all agree: the wrongness of stealing. But, having been alerted by a third party, the social services department was duty bound to follow procedure and investigate.[33] That procedure involved members of the primary healthcare team.

There being no law on corporal punishment as yet in this context, it is possible to argue that the culture and practice of Leo and his family allowed for his caning in response to a serious misdemeanour. Others might say that the physical injury of the child is unacceptable and should be proscribed. The healthcare professionals have a task which is mainly evidential and may be achieved either on the telephone with the investigating social worker or by their attendance at a conference. If so, they might contribute to the decision on further supervision and their own moral perspectives come into play. Should they believe that Leo's father has broken an absolute moral rule they might see this as emotional and physical abuse and recommend accordingly.

One way of conceptualising this kind of problem is to imagine a spectrum of moral 'rightness' rather than an absolute. At one end of the spectrum are acts that we define as completely wrong, and are proscribed by law, such that no consent can be given. Examples include female circumcision which is culturally horrific in the UK, though it retains some adherents in Africa. Statute law here forbids this operation, and arguably lays a moral obligation on UK health professionals to prevent girls being taken overseas to be circumcised.[34] Interestingly enough, in one section, custom and ritual are specifically excluded as allowable reasons for genital mutilation, though 'medical indications' are not.[35] The view that people of a culture, who would normally consider female circumcision, for whatever reason, might consent to such a procedure for their daughter is thus overwhelmed, and ignored.

At the other end of the spectrum is a level of non-physical control of children that all parents of any culture would accept as necessary for moral guidance and learning in general. The difficulty for the child protection authorities is deciding where on the scale Leo's case comes. An objective moral standard does not seem to exist.

Similar problems arise in healthcare every day. For example, is it possible to consent to male circumcision? In the case of a man, who can make an autonomous decision for a therapeutic reason, there seems to be no problem. Where a phimosis can be corrected only by surgery along these lines and the patient is fully informed, then there is no reason not to proceed. Even where there is no therapeutic reason, cultural norms seem to validate the ability to consent, rather along the lines of the 'core values' described above in relation to Jehovah's Witness' decisions. Where the patient is a baby, and the circumcision done for ritual reasons, there may be a greater moral dilemma. Obviously there can be no consent by a baby to a ritual circumcision, but we allow parents to consent for the baby (see Chapter 8). For those cultures in whom this is normal practice, there is no moral dilemma: the procedure grows out of historical or religious custom. Other cultures, or individuals, might regard this as a barbarism. Similar arguments can be advanced for any surgical beautification of minors, for example ear lobe piercing. One route out of this moral impasse could be that consent, at an appropriate stage of development, with full information, freedom of choice and understanding, offers moral justification for a mutilating procedure.

Common law in the UK constrains adult consent as well. One celebrated case held that adults who indulged in extreme sadomasochistic practices could be held to have committed grievous bodily harm.[36] The House of Lords judged that consent could not be given lawfully for extreme sexual practices of this nature, and passed sentence on the participants. Where sexual practices are not quite so extreme, then consent is lawful.[37] Much debate followed this judgement but it is necessary to observe that it is inconsistent with a pre-eminent view of autonomy. Rather, it is aligned with unjustified medical paternalism.

Conclusion

This review of the ethical aspects of consent has demonstrated the pre-eminence of the principle of autonomy. Where there are conflicts with other ethical principles, autonomy generally triumphs, and this the law recognises. Where it does not, the presence of risk of harm to self or others seems to justify the overwhelming of autonomy in a paternalistic manner.

The only other way of considering these matters is through a complete reassessment of what autonomy means. Some philosophers are beginning to do this.

References and notes

1   Berto G (1964) *Incubus*. Penguin, Harmondsworth (translated by Weaver W).
2   O'Brien v Cunard SS Co (1891) **28** *NE:* 266 (*Mass Sup Jud Ct*).
3   Beauchamp TL and Childress J (1994) *Principles of Biomedical Ethics* (4e). Oxford University Press, Oxford, Ch. 3.
4   Malyon D (1998) Transfusion-free treatment of Jehovah's Witnesses: respecting the autonomous patient's rights. *J Med Ethics.* **24**: 302–7. This is a description of their position by an adherent.
5   Code of Practice para 15.15 pursuant to s118[4] Mental Health Act 1983. *See* also General Medical Council (1998) *Seeking Patients' Consent: the ethical considerations.* GMC, London.
6   Re C (Adult: Refusal of Medical Treatment) (1994) **1** *WLR:* 290. Dr Eastman, a psychiatrist and a witness in the case, described what has become known as the 3 stage *Re C* test.
7   When the GP saw Gordon in the general hospital he may have had this scheme in mind when assessing him. Had he any doubt, after discussion with the surgeon, he could seek help from defence bodies and the courts.
8   Pedler M (2000) Mental health and compulsion. *J Mental Health Law.* **3**: 16–27.
9   Hurwitz B (1998) Pressuring Mrs Thomas to accept treatment: a case history. *J Med Ethics.* **24**: 320–1.

10   Rose Gasner M, Maw KL, Feldman GE *et al.* (1999) The use of legal action in New York City to ensure treatment of tuberculosis. *NEJM.* **340**(5): 359–66 and editorial pp. 385–6 (Campion EW).

11   Coker C (2000) Tuberculosis, non-compliance and detention for the public health. *J Med Ethics* **26**: 157–9.

12   *See* Mason JK and McCall Smith RA (1994) *Law and Medical Ethics* (4e) Butterworths, London for a review of this power.

13   Re T (Adult: refusal of medical treatment) (1992) **4** *All ER*: 649, (1992) **9** *BMLR*: 46 (CA).

14   Freeling P and Harris CM (1983) *The Doctor Patient Relationship* (3e). Churchill Livingstone, Edinburgh, Ch. 4.

15   Freeling P and Gask L (1998) Sticks and stones. *BMJ.* **317**: 1028–9.

16   Higgs R (1985) On telling patients the truth. In: *Moral Dilemmas in Modern Medicine.* Oxford University Press, Oxford.

17   Keywood K and Flynn M (2000) Healthcare decision making by, with and for adults with learning difficulties. *Br J Fam Planning.* **26**(1): 58.

18   Bolam v Friern Hospital Management Committee (1957) **2** *All ER*: 118 where a patient suffering fractures after unmodified electroconvulsive treatment did not succeed in establishing negligence against a doctor using this technique because that practice was 'in accordance with the practice accepted by a responsible body of medical men skilled in that particular art'.

19   Bolitho v City and Hackney Health Authority (1997) **4** *All ER*: 771 (HL). This was a medical negligence case of some complexity. Their lordships *inter alia* held that 'responsible' as under *Bolam* meant 'logical' and was not merely a numerical construct.

20   Godwin K (1997) Consumer's understanding of contraceptive efficacy. *Br J Fam Planning* **23**: 45–6.

21   Tate P (1990) *Involving Patients in their Own Care.* Horizons, pp. 21–6.

22. Henderson M (1994) Risk and the doctor–patient relationship. In: R Gillon (ed.) *Principles of Health Care Ethics.* John Wiley & Sons, Chichester.

23   Edwards A and Prior L (1997) Communication about risk – dilemmas for general practitioners. *Br J Gen Pract.* **47**: 739–42.

24   Calman KC and Royston GHD (1997) Risk language and dialects. *BMJ.* **315**: 939–42.

25   Quotation abbreviated.

26   Fahey T and Newton J (1995) Conveying the benefits and risks of treatment. *Br J Gen Pract.* **45**: 339–41.

27   Re F (Mental patient: Sterilisation) (1990) **2** *AC*: 1 *per* Lord Goff.

28   Kennedy I and Grubb A (1994) *Medical Law: text with materials* (2e). Butterworths, London, p. 282.

29   *Parens patriae* is retained for children as the inherent jurisdiction of the court.

30 *T v T* (1988) *Fam*: 2. The judge determined that under this Act even relatives appointed guardians of a patient can give no such consent.

31 General Medical Council (1998) *Seeking Patient's Consent: the ethical considerations.* GMC, London, para 25.

32 McHale JV (1998) Mental incapacity: some proposals for legislative reform. *J Med Ethics.* **24**: 322–7. This article presents the issues clearly.

33 *Children Act* (1989) s47 (1) b: '. . . reasonable cause to suspect that a child . . . is suffering or likely to suffer significant harm'.

34 Prevention of Female Circumcision Act (1985).

35 *Ibid.* s2(2).

36 R v Brown (1993) **2** *All ER*: 75. Consent was unlawful where a group of men used blades and hammers on one another as part of sexual gratification.

37 R v Wilson (1996) **3** *WLR*: 125, CA. Consent was held to be lawful where a man branded his wife's buttocks. The relevant statute is the Offences against the Person Act 1861 as in *Brown* above.

CHAPTER SEVEN

Fertility: making babies – the haves and the have-nots

Summary

Some of the medical and social aspects of human fertility engender complex ethical problems for the GP. There is no hard and fast mandatory rule that can be applied to all cases: sometimes an ethical choice can only be made pragmatically. The problems include:

- Decisions in pregnancy
- Screening in pregnancy
- Failure to conceive
- Assisted fertility
- Fertility restriction
- Abortion
- Surrogacy.

a human being who had not existed a moment ago but who, with the same rights and importance to itself as the rest of humanity, would live and create others in its own image ... Whence, wherefore had it come, and who was it?[1]

Introduction

The medical aspects of human fertility involve doctors in many and varied ethical debates. Not all are relevant to general practice at the moment, although some may become so in the future. In these debates, it is important to appreciate the ideals to which we subscribe as a society; it would be difficult to argue against any effort made to ensure the natural birth of a healthy normal child to caring and well-adjusted parents following an uncomplicated pregnancy. The welfare of the future child as well as the mother is borne in mind; sometimes it is the moral necessity to achieve this balance which perplexes the doctor.

The first main problem can arise with the newly pregnant woman. She will be encouraged to discuss with her GP her lifestyle during pregnancy, what tests and examinations will be recommended, and choices for delivery. If she does not comply with reasonable evidence-based medical advice in spite of understanding the risks, her health and that of her baby may suffer. The GP is likely to be concerned about her choices, but equally, has a duty to respect them as being made by an autonomous individual.

There are two other main problems with fertility that we shall discuss in this chapter: *failure to conceive* and *unwanted pregnancy*. The GP is liable to face complex ethical dilemmas in both these areas and needs to be aware of the ethical and legal issues of assisted fertility and abortion.

Other areas are of increasing importance due to advances in medical technology: postcoital contraception, antenatal screening for fetal abnormality and surrogacy.

Decisions in pregnancy

In the past, most women delivered their babies at home, under the care of the community midwife. The GP would not necessarily be called upon to attend if the birth progressed normally. A hospital confinement was reserved for those mothers who were judged to need more intensive medical supervision.

Now, most babies are born in hospital and home deliveries are rare in most parts of the country. Many GPs have little continuing experience of intrapartum care; naturally they are reluctant to take on the responsibility if a patient wishes to have her baby at home. Community midwives have the expertise, but the duty of care to the patient rests with the GP as well. Some women are insistent on a home delivery, and against any form of medical intervention in labour or at delivery.

Ruth is 44 years old, and pregnant for the sixth time. Her last confinement eight years ago was at home, and was normal. Since then she has had two miscarriages. She and her husband are delighted that this pregnancy is progressing well. They have refused antenatal screening: for religious reasons, they could not contemplate termination. Ruth wants another home birth. Sarah, the community midwife is unhappy about this and has tried unsuccessfully to dissuade Ruth. Sarah asks the GP to support her with Ruth: 'you might have more influence', she says.

There are several strands to consider in this dilemma:

- outcome for the child
- outcome for the mother
- role of the father in decision making
- professional integrity of the midwife
- role of the GP in decision making
  - paternalism
  - coercion
  - respecting the patient's autonomy.

Current medical opinion would endorse the choice of hospital rather than home delivery for Ruth, with the probability of a better outcome for both mother and child. This information may not carry any weight with Ruth for whom statistics may be meaningless and the probability only conjecture on the part of her GP and the midwife. She feels that she and her baby will be better off at home.

We do not know what the baby's father's opinion is. He will be either fully supportive of Ruth or merely acquiescent. No doubt he would have expressed his disagreement by now if he had been against the idea of a home birth. We do know, however, that the midwife is unsure about taking responsibility for the confinement – which she will have to do if Ruth continues to insist. Sarah has a duty of care to Ruth. Is it right that Ruth should impose her will on

Sarah, against sound advice, and risk compromising Sarah's professional integrity? Does Ruth have a reciprocal duty to someone in Sarah's position?

Certainly, the GP has a duty to Ruth. Does he also have a duty to the expected child? Maybe there is statistical evidence that the chances of a good outcome for both mother and child are reduced by conducting the confinement in the home rather than in a hospital where expertise and equipment are to hand if needed. Would the statistical difference be affected by Ruth's negative attitude to medical intervention? She would probably argue that if she were to be supported in her choice of having the baby at home, she would be happier and therefore would have a better chance of a normal confinement.

An attempt by the GP to *persuade*[2] Ruth, as the midwife has asked, would need the GP to adopt a paternalistic approach. As Sarah has suggested, he would be using his position of power and control to subordinate Ruth's autonomy to current medical opinion in the expectation of a better outcome. The GP would be supporting the opinion of the midwife, a professional colleague. This course of action by the GP may also be his duty to his patient and her child.

How do you respond to Sarah's request?

Ethical problems concerning a woman's self-determination can arise towards the end of pregnancy, perhaps when an unforeseen complication arises. This may mean that the patient's prior choice of delivery needs to be renegotiated. The choice – perhaps a home delivery, perhaps refusing medical intervention – may now be medically untenable, unwise or even dangerous.

On seeking to register as a new patient at a local NHS practice, S, who was 36 weeks pregnant, was diagnosed with pre-eclampsia and advised that she needed to be admitted to hospital for an induced delivery. S fully understood the potential risks but rejected the advice as she wanted her baby to be born naturally.[3]

The GP in this actual case was faced with a very real moral dilemma. Here was a new patient, at a late stage in pregnancy, with a medical condition threatening not only her own life but also that of her unborn child. The recommended medical intervention was likely to avert the danger to both of them – and she was refusing that intervention. Her insistence on a 'natural birth' seemed most unreasonable: the odds were against a good outcome.

The more advanced a pregnancy, and the more likely that a normal viable child will be delivered, the more morally repugnant is the notion that the child's life be put at risk at the will of the mother, in order to protect her rights. If we accept that the life of the 36-week-old foetus has an important intrinsic value which ought to be protected, that concept needs to be balanced against the mother's right to decide what happens to her own body.

Unfortunately, the law currently gives us little option, provided the mother is competent to make her own decision. Any intervention without consent would be deemed to be a criminal assault – as was decided by the Court of Appeal in the case of S. The court held that the unborn child's interests did not prevail over the patient's right to refuse treatment and the treatment given to S amounted to a battery and was unlawful.[4] The right of choice for a mentally competent adult patient to refuse medical intervention is absolute in law.

> This right of choice is not limited to decisions which others might regard as sensible. It exists not withstanding that the reasons for making the choice are rational, irrational, unknown or even non-existent.[5]

It is to be hoped that in general practice such a situation would occur only very rarely. However, it is vitally important that the moral questions that it raises are explored. It could be that the GP would feel on morally sound ground if he brought to bear all means of persuasion, coercion, paternalism and control into discussion with his patient in order to influence her decision. The moral justification for such tactics, however overtly unsound in terms of respect for her autonomy, would be the preservation not only of her life but that of the child.

Dworkin identifies the underlying intuition that governs the argument – that of the creative investment in human life which progresses throughout pregnancy giving the foetus an increasing *value* as term approaches. He is describing the debate on abortion, but the basic premise applies equally well in this context.[6]

Screening in pregnancy

The prospect of 'screening out' all fetal abnormalities is an ethically contentious issue. It is only possible to do this with certain conditions at the moment, and even then, not always with absolute certainty. Advances in techniques of screening in pregnancy continue at a rapid pace, and have, quite rightly and predictably, initiated widespread concern and discussion of the moral rectitude of the process (*see* Chapter 4).

A good example is screening for Down's syndrome using ultrasound measurement of nuchal translucency. When this was first developed, there was an expectation that the rate of births of Down's syndrome babies would go down dramatically, the cost to society of caring for these individuals would be cut, and the savings could be put to other uses.

This expectation was ill-founded. The calculations did not take into consideration two important factors: the demise of possible affected foetuses in early pregnancy, and the number of mothers unwilling either to take part in the screening programme or to rely on statistics to govern a decision to terminate a pregnancy.

At the very least, the ethical basis for such an expectation in healthcare planning is dubious. Reliance on a woman to decide to abort her foetus on the grounds that it *might statistically* be born with Down's syndrome is a mechanistic assumption. One woman faced with an increased likelihood of 4% of this happening may choose to ask for a further invasive test, which in itself carries a risk of miscarriage. Another with an increased risk of 8% may decide against a further test, being unwilling to risk a viable pregnancy. Other women, offered the test as routine, will decide against it as they would not consider termination on such grounds.

The principle underlying the concept of screening for a condition such as Down's syndrome is that the birth of such children is not only undesirable, but that it should in some way be prevented. This could be perceived as the beginning of the slippery slope towards the practice of eugenics, where only 'high quality' foetuses are allowed to survive. It is not surprising that the principle of eugenics, or selective breeding, should have come to be regarded with abhorrence in the second half of the last century. What started as a desire to give parents more of a surety that the children born to them would approach 'the norm' in society, whatever that might be, is now feared by some as a progression towards the production of 'designer' babies (*see* Chapter 4).

It appears to those with a disability, whether congenital, inherited or acquired, that subsumed in this principle is the idea that society values them less as human beings than so-called 'normal' people. This attitude begs the question of whether it is a misfortune for them that they have been born. Someone who is born with a disability, or the potential for one, already exists, and is unlikely to say that they wished they had never had an existence.

The idea of a 'genetic lottery' has been described by Holtug in an article discussing the ethics of genetic enhancement. He points out that each individual is born with a set of genes which is unique to that individual, a set which he has not chosen for himself. It is this lack of choice on which Holtug bases his idea of the lottery. In this genetic lottery lies each person's future, with the potential for health or disease.[7] In accordance with Rawls, if in that lottery some people have drawn less beneficially than others, this does not mean that society should allow an egalitarian principle of justice to pass them by. In Rawls' ideal society, *each* person's well-being will depend on what he terms 'social cooperation'.[8]

The question of screening will arise where there is a family history of a disabling inherited condition, or where a prospective parent knows that they carry the gene for such a condition. Couples in this predicament will be referred to a genetics clinic that has the necessary expertise to inform and counsel them. The GP will only be drawn in if they remain undecided whether to try to conceive or not. A dispassionate viewpoint is imperative; it must be, after all, the couple's own informed decision. Bias or prejudice play no part in the interchange.

Whatever the initial reason for a discussion between the patient and GP on antenatal screening, the GP has a duty to describe the process and to make sure that the patient understands all the implications of such screening. Without this part of the discussion, the patient may initiate a process the implications of which she does not really understand. She needs to be prepared to face up to some of the unexpected and difficult decisions she may be asked to make.

On the other hand, some patients are particularly well informed on the implications of screening.

> Tanya is a single mother with a young daughter. She is preg-
> nant again. She has come to book in for antenatal care. She
> asks for antenatal screening for foetal abnormality, and says
> that if this shows that the foetus is a boy, she will ask for a ter-
> mination. Her brother and a young cousin are haemophiliacs,
> and she has experienced first hand the effect this has had on
> their lives and the anguish for the family. She does not want
> knowingly to inflict the same on another child.

It would appear that Tanya's main reason for asking for screening is to discover the sex of the foetus. This is important to her, in the light of her family experience. Her reason to ask for a termination if the foetus is male is a strong one. We know that support for such a request would be untenable in our society had it been based on cultural demands: the importance in some cultures to raise sons rather than daughters.

The dilemma that Tanya presents is that of any woman who knows that she is likely to be the carrier of a serious X-linked disease.[9] We could argue that a screening test performed primarily to identify the level of risk for foetal abnormality which *incidentally* provides information on the sex of the foetus can *also* be used to provide information of the level of risk of sex-linked disorders. Whether such information can then be used as the reason for a request for legal abortion is another matter (*see* below).

Failure to conceive

Some couples choose to remain childless, but there are many others for whom childlessness is involuntary. The amount of distress that this causes varies between different couples, but also between the man and the woman in the partnership.

William and his wife Yasmin are new patients to the practice. William comes for a routine new patient check. He tells the GP that this is his second marriage; he has two children from his former marriage. Yasmin has no children, and is desperately keen to conceive: this has not happened and she wants fertility treatment. William definitely does not want the responsibility of any more children. He asks the GP not to refer Yasmin to the fertility centre however much she pleads.

Any discussion on the moral dilemma presented by this story is theoretical. A fertility centre would be unlikely to accept this couple for treatment unless both husband and wife agreed that this was what they wanted. We are left with the question of Yasmin's right to have a child which conflicts with her husband's right not to father a child, and which of these rights 'trumps' the other.

Assisted fertility

It is possible to help many infertile couples to achieve a successful pregnancy, thanks to increasingly refined methods of assisted fertility. The first medical contact made by such couples will normally be the GP. They will be asking for investigations and information, to explore reasons for their difficulty and to help them to access treatment.

There is a primary assumption that infertility is a medical rather than a social problem. It is on this assumption that the provision of fertility treatment on the NHS rests, as well as the necessary involvement of the gatekeeper – the GP. If this were not so, all assisted fertility programmes would be funded by the couple.

The second assumption is that everyone has a right to start a family.[10] Natural conception has no restrictions placed on it by society. However, assisted conception – in vitro fertilisation (IVF) – cannot take place unless both prospective parents have had a satisfactory assessment of their desirability as parents medically and, more controversially, socially.

The third assumption is that age, in particular maternal age, is no barrier to assisted fertility. Many couples choose to start their families later in life when they have reached a certain point in their careers which assures financial stability. This may have a deleterious effect on fertility, which tends to reduce with age. The older couple may be in a new relationship where they desire a child of that union. This means that older women now have the expectation that, if natural conception has not occurred, with medical intervention they can still bear a child. Unfortunately they may not be aware that the percentage success rate of assisted conception declines with advancing age.

Fourthly, medical problems such as pelvic disease or azoospermia are now surmountable with the advanced specialist techniques available to couples, and couples can become parents of children with part or even no genetic link with them (*see* p. 159 for surrogacy).

In summary, the main ethical issues are:

- access to resources
- screening of social and medical history
- effects of age
- use of special medical techniques.

Access to resources

Ethical principle of justice

Fertility centres are increasing in number across the country, expertise is widely available for all but the most specialised techniques, and standards of treatment are monitored. Overall success rates are variable, but this may be a reflection on the type of patient accepted by different centres for treatment: the chance of a successful outcome is higher in some patient groups than in others. Capacity appears to be such that the waiting list for self-funding couples is either very short or non-existent.

It is the question of funding that poses the greatest resource problem and the resulting ethical dilemma. Few couples are in the financial position of being able to fund for themselves even one course of treatment in total, and more would be out of the question. NHS funding is more easily forthcoming in some areas than in others, and in some parts of the UK than in others. Waiting lists for treatment tend to be very long. Some patients are accepted onto NHS fertility programmes only to find that not all the treatment will be funded – the drugs necessary to support the intervention are not. They will then approach the GP for an NHS prescription for the drugs, which may or may not be forthcoming.[11]

GPs now find themselves involved in daily decisions on allocation of resources, an increasing number of which involve infertile couples seeking help (*see* Chapter 10). Several questions require answers, each with a pronounced ethical dimension, but *only* if it is agreed that assisted fertility *ought* to be provided by the NHS.

---

1 Should NHS treatment be available to *all* couples?
2 If not, on what grounds will couples be accepted or refused by the GP for referral?
3 Should all the treatment be free to patients or should they pay for the drugs themselves?
4 How many courses of treatment ought to be provided on the NHS?

Screening of social and medical history

Ethical principles of autonomy and justice

> The laws which, in many countries on the Continent, forbid marriage unless the parties can show that they have the means of supporting the family, do not exceed the legitimate powers of the state: and whether such laws be expedient or not ... they are not objectionable as violations of liberty.[12]

Mill made this statement in 1859. His philosophical view of what constituted liberty then would be severely criticised now. Yet his words are paraphrased in the Human Fertilisation and Embryology Act (1990). Section 13(5) states that 'a woman shall not be provided with treatment services unless account has been taken of the welfare of any child who may be born as a result of the treatment (including the need of that child for a father) and of any other child who might be affected by the birth.'

The implication here is that the 'parties' applying for treatment must include a father who fulfils his parental role in the social as well as the biological sense. If they cannot demonstrate this, treatment under the Act is denied – in effect, forbidden. In addition, it could be said that the 'welfare' of the child would depend on the financial status of the family into which it is born. If the applicants are unable to support a child in the material sense, in theory, they could be denied treatment.[13]

The moral argument for such restriction of liberty as expressed by both Mill and the 1990 Act is based on concern for the welfare of any future children. In both examples, Mill in 1859 and those who constructed the wording of the Act in 1990 considered it to be the State's duty to legislate on these lines, restricting the liberty of the individual in order to favour the establishment of a sound base for 'good' families.

If we examine this in more detail, the natural conception of children is fundamentally different from conception that involves a third party – the fertility treatment centre. The prevention of conception is normally a free choice made by the individual, either by abstention or by contraception. Here we are dealing not with the prevention of conception but with the refusal to aid conception by artificial means.

We know that there is now a possibility for preimplantation screening where, out of a group of embryos, those that are potentially 'imperfect' are rejected, and only those seemingly potentially healthy are implanted. The ethical argument is clear: *choosing* to implant an imperfect embryo would be ethically wrong as it could result in the birth of a disadvantaged individual. Those responsible would not have considered the welfare of the future child.[14]

Likewise, if the fertility centre considered that a treatment was against the interests of the future child, and thereby against the interests of society as a whole, that a child born as a result of such active intervention would be disadvantaged in some substantial way, then it could be ethically justified in refusing an intervention likely to bring about the creation of such a child.

The GP is well placed to know patients' social backgrounds as well as their medical histories. The Human Fertilisation and Embryology Authority's Code of Practice (1995) recognises the GP as an important source of information and requires centres to make use of this as well as interviewing the applicants personally. 'Centres should seek to satisfy themselves that the GP of each prospective parent knows of no reason why either of them might not be suitable for the treatment to be offered. This would include anything which might adversely affect the welfare of any resulting child.'[15] It is the 'welfare of the resulting child' which is paramount.

How is this to be interpreted by the GP? The difficulty lies with the use of wording which is non-specific regarding suitability for parenthood and adverse effects on the child. The fertility centre will be relying on objectivity on the part of the GP, yet it is possible for the GP's response to questions on the form to be weighted in some way, depending on the GP's societal attitude and moral stance. How far a negative view on a particular person's desirability as a parent by the GP would affect acceptance for treatment by a centre is unclear, and ought to be taken in context, together with any other relevant factors.[16]

Effects of age

Ethical principle of justice

Infertility in the younger woman, whether primary or secondary, is often due to a well-defined medical problem; such a patient would not be rejected for fertility treatment on the grounds of age. However, advancing maternal age is an important consideration for several reasons, not all of them based on medical evidence. There is strong evidence that there is an increased risk of fetal loss in older women. In one population study in Denmark, it was found that at age 42 more than half of all pregnancies intended to reach term ended with foetal loss. The comparable risk in the 25–29 years age group is very much lower, and the risk appears to rise sharply over the age of 35 years.[17]

Effective control over fertility in younger women, who choose to delay their first pregnancy until they are in their 30s, may now be having an adverse effect on their chances of achieving that pregnancy and sustaining it to term. If natural conception eludes them as they get older, many of them will be hoping to obtain fertility treatment through the NHS. The question has already been posed earlier in this chapter: should all couples be able to have treatment, and if not, what factors ought to govern their acceptance or refusal? Accepting all ages for a treatment for which there is a fixed budget means that those younger women, who perhaps have a better chance of success, are disadvantaged by having to join a longer waiting list for treatment. In view of the reduced likelihood of success in older women, should there be an age beyond which the NHS will not fund treatment? Younger women would be better served by the system and there would be a better rate of success. Scarce resources would not be 'wasted'.

The deontological view would reject this as unethical – there is a duty to each and every person which would be compromised if selection on grounds of age were in place. The utilitarian would take a different stance: the common good would be better served by concentrating resources where most benefit is likely to be derived. The latter view is the one often taken by the health authorities that draw up the list of qualifying factors for acceptance onto NHS fertility programmes.

If we turn to non-NHS self-funded treatment, there have been much-publicised successful cases involving women in their sixties having fertility treatment in other European countries. As far as is known, this has not happened in this country. Setting an upper maternal age limit for treatment would supposedly be based on the estimated welfare of the future child. Not only would such treatment be technically more difficult but it could be argued that a child of an aged mother with a relatively short life expectancy would be at some sort of disadvantage. This can be disproved by the examples of children being brought up by grandparents, as well as by appreciation of the material benefit and social advantage to a child of older financially secure parents.

Use of special medical techniques

Ethical principle of autonomy

The practical aspects of specialised techniques are clearly not within the remit of the GP. Nevertheless, it is important that the GP is aware of the range of services which are available in particular circumstances and of some of the main hazards involved. A couple may have been to the fertility centre and come away with some of their questions as yet unanswered. Although the GP cannot expect to be able to inform on the detail, he has a responsibility to reassure himself that the couple is in a position to make an informed decision on treatment; this is a responsibility shared with the medical staff at the centre, although for the GP it will be to a lesser degree. A choice between two options for treatment may have been offered to them and they have difficulty in making a decision on which option to choose. Discussion with the GP may help them to come to an autonomous decision providing the GP remains impartial as well as supportive.

Role of the Human Fertilisation and Embryology Authority (HFEA)

The HFEA was set up in 1990 in response to the recommendations of the Warnock Committee of Inquiry.[18] The Warnock Committee was asked particularly to consider the social, ethical and legal implications of recent advances in this important area of medicine. The Human Fertilisation and Embryology Act (1990) regulates infertility treatment that involves the use of donated gametes as well as IVF. There is no statutory regulation of other forms of fertility treatment, such as ovarian stimulation or artificial insemination by husband (AIH).

The HFEA has several functions under the 1990 Act. Those of primary importance to GPs and their patients seeking infertility treatment are:

- to license treatment services, the storage of gametes and embryos, and research on embryos
- to maintain a code of practice as guidance for the proper conduct of activities carried out under a licence.

Under this ruling, once a fertility clinic has been licensed for treatment services it is bound to abide by the HFEA's code of practice, which is updated from time to time. If it does not, it runs the risk of the licence being withdrawn. This assures patients, not only of the maintenance of good clinical practice, but also of protection of confidentiality, counselling and information.

As we have seen earlier, the code of practice aims to ensure as far as is possible the welfare of the future child by requiring the fertility clinic to conduct 'a fair and unprejudiced assessment of [people's] situation and needs, which should be conducted with the skill and sensitivity appropriate to the delicacy of the case and the wishes and feelings of those involved'.[19] It is not difficult to predict where ethical conflicts arise during such an assessment: some of these have already been the subject of court cases, media publicity and public debate. Anyone with a criminal record, history of prostitution,[20] a significant psychiatric or psychosexual history, or a medical condition likely to reduce life expectancy, might be considered unsuitable for treatment, as might be a single woman with no male partner or an HIV positive person. It is important to recognise, however, that opinions on such restrictions are continually changing. It was reported that an HIV positive couple were rejected for treatment in 1991 yet a woman, also HIV positive, was accepted in 1996. This change could reflect the advance in knowledge and treatment outcomes of this hitherto untreatable condition, hence a better prospect for the family and future child.[21] When examining the ethics of access to treatment we need to separate the question of *primary access* of infertile people to treatment for their infertility from their *access to NHS-funded treatment* where the rules are more restricting and rationing decisions come into play.

If we consider the infertile people who seek treatment from fertility clinics, all of them will have the same end in view – the birth of a child. The HFEA has decided that there should be a screening mechanism which will exclude all those with characteristics which some consider unsuitable in a parent. This decision has not yet been successfully challenged legally: is it *ethically* sound?

---

1   Ought fertility treatment to be available to all?
2   If there ought to be some exclusions, what characteristics would guarantee refusal to treat?

Fertility restriction

Those who do not wish to produce a child will either practice efficient contraception or apply for termination of pregnancy. There is an indeterminate area between these two possibilities: so-called postcoital contraception which although termed 'contraception' is designed to prevent successful implantation of a fertilised ovum, i.e. postconception.

Contraception

In most cases that concern the provision of contraception, the consultation is straightforward. The patient has decided that that is what she needs, and the GP will discuss with her the various options so that she can make an informed choice. The GP's duty will have been fulfilled and the patient's autonomy respected. Even with an underage patient, providing the GP adheres to the rules of 'Gillick competence' the same applies (*see* Chapter 8).

Some GPs have a conscientious objection to providing contraception. They are nevertheless duty bound to direct the patient to another GP or to a family planning service where advice and treatment will be provided. Failure to do this would be tantamount to applying pressure on the patient not to use contraception. Although many women would be able to find an alternative source of advice on their own, there will still be some who are not and need further information and help.

Alma is 22 years old and has three children by three different men. The youngest child is 8 months old. She met her latest boyfriend, Bob, after he came out of prison recently, where he had served a brief term for possession of drugs. Bob's history came to the GP via the health visitor, who has expressed some concern about Alma's maternal capabilities on several occasions. Alma had an IUD fitted after the last child. It has been trouble-free, but now she has come to the GP asking for it to be taken out. She and Bob want a child.

We have already discussed the question of what makes a suitable parent, and whether there are some people who appear to be so unsuitable that the welfare of the future child is likely to be compromised. If the GP removes the IUD as Alma desires, and Alma conceives with Bob as a result, can we make any assumptions as to the quality of life of the new member of this family? Further, will the quality of life for the existing children be affected by the addition of another child? Is it fair if society makes such predictions and judgements? Can the GP justify a refusal to comply with Alma's request, perhaps on the grounds of mental and physical strain on Alma herself inflicted by another pregnancy and birth, another baby in what seems to be an already stressed family?

> What ought the GP to do?

Postcoital contraception

The language is ambiguous when it refers to postcoital *contraception* as preventing the implantation of the fertilised ovum. In theory, a chemical or mechanical treatment which has this effect is an abortifacient. In practice, the law has decided that anything which has the effect of ending a pregnancy *before* implantation could not be referred to as procuring a miscarriage, and therefore is not illegal and does not need to be covered by the Abortion Act.

If, however, an IUD were to be fitted *after* implantation had occurred, it would bring about a miscarriage. It is unlikely that the doctor could be certain that this was the case, and therefore unlikely that he could be convicted.[22] The *ethical* consideration remains in place even as the legal threat is removed.

There are some GPs who would have a moral difficulty about prescribing postcoital contraception. It is important that this is made clear to patients in good time: there ought not to be any delay for treatment for women attending their GP for postcoital contraception.[23]

Abortion

The philosophical debate on the rights and wrongs of abortion is cast at two extremes. The argument that under no circumstances can the life of the foetus be ended is at one extreme. At the other extreme is the argument that the mother's autonomy is paramount and abortion can occur at any time – pro life versus pro choice. In reality, the debate hinges on the understanding of 'the right to

life'. We can start with Aristotle's definition of a human being as a
'rational being', rationality implying certain cognitive and psychological capacities which are necessary for self-determination, or
autonomy. If this is what we mean by 'personhood', a person having an intrinsic moral value, then do we agree that only persons
have rights, that they are the only ones with a right to life?

Using this train of deduction, it would be difficult to argue for the
right to life of a foetus overriding that of the mother. Yet after conception has taken place, each embryo or foetus is a *potential* person.
How does this *potentiality* affect the right to life argument? Thomson, in her essay on abortion, puts into the balance the 'right to life'
of the unborn child and the 'right to decide what happens to one's
own body' of the pregnant woman.[24] She accepts that the potential
child has a right not to be killed, but this right is not an *absolute* right
based on the *mandatory* ethical principle that it is fundamentally
wrong to kill someone. There are particular situations giving rise to
an unwanted pregnancy, or arising during a pregnancy, where the
mother's rights can morally be allowed to override those of her
foetus. Abortion in these situations would be based on an *elective*
principle, where there are convincing arguments on either side.
Foot has drawn the distinction between mandatory and elective
principles.[25] Danger to the mother's life if pregnancy continued, the
substantial risk of fetal malformation such as anencephaly, or as in
Tanya's case, haemophilia if the foetus was male, and pregnancy as a
result of rape are all situations where an elective ethical principle
would support abortion.

On the other hand it would be difficult to support ethically an
abortion performed for social convenience – a holiday, or a new job.

Carol, her husband and their 12-year-old daughter have just
moved into a new house. She has a good job, the income from
which supports most of the new mortgage and her daughter's
private schooling. She had a prolonged period of depression
some years ago needing inpatient treatment, at a time when
her husband suffered short-term redundancy. Carol has missed
a period and home pregnancy testing confirms her worst fears –
she is pregnant. She comes to see her GP in a great deal of
distress asking for a termination.

The law in this country now allows abortion under certain circumstances. Although abortion seems to be strictly regulated by the Abortion Act (1967),[26] nevertheless, it is perceived by some as allowing 'abortion on demand' for many women. If it is to be interpreted in the widest sense, it is possible to claim on statistical grounds that a pregnancy which has not yet reached 12 weeks' gestation carries more risk to the mother's health than an abortion at that stage. It is therefore possible to comply with the law in recommending an abortion before 12 weeks under Section 1(1)(a) by using this comparative exercise.[27]

If we examine Carol's request purely from the *legal* point of view, she would fulfil the requirements under Section 1(1)(a) of the 1967 Act. This states that it is not an offence if a pregnancy is terminated where it has not exceeded 24 weeks and its continuance 'would involve risk, greater than if the pregnancy were terminated, of injury to the physical or mental health of the pregnant woman or any existing children of her family.'

Yet we might have concerns about the *ethical* justification for recommending a termination in this instance. As with many of the dilemmas that face the GP, the outcome will depend on a balancing exercise. The following progression of thought may go through the GP's mind:

- Carol is in the early weeks of pregnancy
- if the pregnancy continues the family may suffer financially – although this cannot be predicted with certainty
- she is distressed – today.

Is the inconvenience of the pregnancy the reason for her request for termination?

But also

- Carol has a history of a significant depressive illness
- there may be a recurrence if pregnancy continues – although this cannot be predicted with certainty
- she is distressed – this distress may continue.

Is the anxiety about that particular sequence of events the reason for her request for termination?

Having fulfilled the legal requirements, is there any ethical argument that can be used to support Carol's termination? Or is there a lack of consistency between the law and ethics?

There was a considerable amount of public concern following a case which came to the courts recently at the possibility that a GP might try to impose his or her views or to use undue influence to dissuade a woman from seeking an abortion. In this particular case, *Barr v Matthews* (1999), the GP had a conscientious objection to abortion. The patient consulted the GP in early pregnancy and was not referred for an abortion as she wished, nor was she referred to another doctor. The patient lost the case against the GP because the evidence before the court was conflicting. The GP stated that she did not consider that the patient had legal grounds for an abortion. It appeared that the patient was unaware of the GP's moral stance. The judge in this case expressed concern that the GP's approach may have been coloured by her moral and religious views. As has been mentioned, some doctors may have a firmly held belief that abortion is wrong and are unwilling to have anything to do with the process. Nevertheless, the GP has a duty to the patient that is made clear thus:

> If you feel that your beliefs might affect the treatment you provide, you must explain this to patients, and tell them of their right to see another doctor.[28]

Clearly it would be wrong for a GP to refuse even to see a patient who was asking for termination: the patient consults the doctor in good faith, and if that first doctor is unable or unwilling to help, another avenue must be provided. Equally, it would be wrong for the GP to try to impose his or her own views on a patient, however strongly they were held. An impartial view is essential in this difficult area, and the patient needs to be assisted towards her own autonomous decision.

Dora is a shy, rather insecure, 17-year-old. She has missed a period and her friends at school have helped her pluck up courage to see the GP as she thinks she might be pregnant. She is scared, and knows she does not want this pregnancy. Her family's GP is one of the male partners – but Dora would rather see the only female partner in the practice. She makes an urgent appointment with her, not revealing the true reason.

This story is a familiar one to many GPs. Every week, a GP will see at least one young girl in this position, or one very similar. The outcome is not always the same: after counselling, some will be referred for termination, some will continue with the pregnancy with support from family or friends. Yet what if Dora, unbeknown to herself, has chosen to consult the only doctor in the partnership with a conscientious objection to abortion? No doubt she will be nonplussed by the GP's reaction, however sensitively she is dealt with. Her courage and determination will need to carry her over yet another hurdle when she has to explain her position yet again to another doctor with different views.

1 Does the practice have a duty to inform patients of the conscientious objection of any of the GPs or nurses?
2 If so, how can this best be done?

Medicinal abortion is now possible using mifepristone. This has little relevance in general practice at the moment but may be more relevant in the future. There has been a recommendation that this particular abortifacient be used in GP surgeries, with proper supervision. The treatment does not require hospitalisation and patients would benefit.

However, under the current law this is not possible, and the law would have to be changed. The problem lies with the necessity for approval by the Secretary of State of a place or class of places where the abortion takes place. The course of medicinal treatment carries over several days and the patient may complete the abortion in her own home or a place other than the GP's surgery. Technically, the Secretary of State would have to approve all the places that the woman might visit between the administration of mifepristone and the eventual abortion – clearly an impractical suggestion.

Surrogacy

This is an aspect of human fertility that has probably been practised since biblical times.[29] According to the Warnock Report it is 'the practice whereby one woman carries a child for another with the intention that the child should be handed over after birth'.[30]

The main ethical concern with a surrogacy arrangement is that it could be regarded as treating someone (the surrogate mother) as a means to an end (the provision of a child for someone else), an arrangement which flouts the Kantian principle of the 'categorical imperative'. As Kant states, man 'exists as an end in himself, not merely as a means for arbitrary use by this or that will.'[31] Another important ethical concern is with the payment of the surrogate mother. This would have the effect of regarding the child as a 'package' to be purchased for a certain price, which is a morally repugnant idea.[32] Commercial contracts between a surrogate mother and a commissioning couple are illegal in this country and unenforceable, although the legislation does allow payment of the surrogate mother's reasonable expenses.[33] There is a body of opinion which views this arrangement as exploitation of the surrogate, who is performing a service for the commissioning couple and ought to be paid a proper amount for her work, not merely her expenses.

At any one time, there is a possibility that a GP will be providing antenatal care for a woman carrying a baby for another, unaware of the arrangement. The surrogate mother may have found surrogacy a useful source of income for a while, her 'reasonable expenses' being more than she could expect otherwise. Her general health and lifestyle may be less than perfect, and unlikely to improve during pregnancy.

Elaine is married with four children from the marriage. She is a heavy smoker with a history of genital warts. She has already had one surrogate pregnancy and handed the baby over to the commissioning couple. The current pregnancy is also the result of another private surrogacy arrangement. Now 13 weeks pregnant, the commissioning couple have pulled out, and she wants an abortion.

This illustrates only one of many ethical problems which surrogacy may produce for the GP. It is impossible to predict the future of surrogacy and whether it is a practice that will become more widespread. Any relaxation of the restrictions currently in place under the Surrogacy Act is unlikely, in particular, the restriction of payments to surrogates. The view that this discourages the treatment of babies as commodities rather than human beings will prevail.

Conclusion

Fertility – the process of reproduction – is a natural phenomenon. Ideally, it requires medical supervision rather than medical intervention. Ethical problems only arise when the natural function is interrupted, involuntarily by failure to conceive or voluntarily by unwanted conception. The ways in which these problems are resolved have attracted considerable public and political interest, such that an understanding of the legal aspects is as important as the ethical principles involved.

References and notes

1   Tolstoy LN (1978 revision by Edmonds R) *Anna Karenina*. Penguin, London, p.749. Tolstoy is describing Levin's thoughts on the birth of his son.
2   Implying an intention to coerce Ruth.
3   St George's Healthcare NHS Trust v S, R v Collins and others, ex parte S (1998) **3** *All ER*: 673.
4   R v Collins, ex p S (1998) (CA).
5   Lord Donaldson in Re T (Adult: refusal of treatment) (1992) **4** *All ER*.
6   Dworkin R (1994) *Life's Dominion*. Vintage Books, New York.
7   Holtug N (1999) Does justice require genetic enhancements? *J Med Ethics.* **25**(2): 137–43.
8   Rawls J (1972) *A Theory of Justice*. Oxford University Press, Oxford, pp. 100–8.
9   McGowan R (1999) Beyond the disorder: one parent's reflection on genetic counselling. *J Med Ethics.* **25**(2): 195–9.

10   Human Rights Act 1998 Article 12 which states the 'right to marry and found a family'. However, it does not indicate the means by which a family can be produced or whether the right includes the use of technology.

11   It is expected that this anomaly will cease to exist with the new configuration of primary healthcare.

12   Mill JS (1962) On liberty. In: M Warnock (ed.) *Utilitarianism*. Harper-Collins, Glasgow, p. 242.

13   Freeman M (1998) Medically Assisted Reproduction. In: I Kennedy and A Grubb (eds) *Principles of Medical Law*. Oxford University Press, Oxford, pp. 564–6.

14   For further discussion of the ethics of this situation see Draper H and Chadwick R Beware! Preimplantation genetic diagnosis may solve some old problems but it also raises new ones. *J Med Ethics*. **25**(2): 114–20.

15   HFEA Code of Practice (1995) 3.24.

16   These are listed in the HFEA Code of Practice (1995) 3.16 and 3.17.

17   Anderson A-M, Wohlfart J, Christens J *et al*. (2000) Maternal age and foetal loss: population based register linkage study. *BMJ*. **320**: 1708–12.

18   DoH (1984) *Report of the Committee of Inquiry into Human Fertilisation and Embryology*. HMSO, London.

19   HFEA Code of Practice (1995).

20   R v Ethical Committee of St Mary's Hospital (Manchester), ex p H (1988) **1** *FLR*: 512. The applicant for IVF treatment was rejected because of a history of prostitution offences.

21   Freeman M (1998) Medically Assisted Reproduction. In: I Kennedy and A Grubb (eds) *Principles of Medical Law*. Oxford University Press, Oxford, p. 569.

22   Grubb A (1998) Abortion. In: I Kennedy and A Grubb (eds) *Principles of Medical Law*. Oxford University Press, Oxford, pp. 613–16.

23   This situation changes with the availability of postcoital contraceptive pills 'over the counter'.

24   Thomson JJ (1977) A defence of abortion. In: RM Dworkin (ed.) *The Philosophy of Law*. Oxford University Press, Oxford.

25   Foot P (1970) *Morality and Art* (Henrietta Herz lecture). Proceedings of the British Academy, London.

26   The Abortion Act 1967 was amended and made more liberal by Section 37 of the Human Fertilisation and Embryology Act 1991.

27   The legal requirements which must be satisfied before an abortion is recommended are listed on Certificate A Form HSA1 (revised 1991). This certificate is to be completed by two registered medical practitioners, having formed an opinion 'in good faith' that one or more of these requirements is fulfilled, before an abortion is carried out. A confusion can arise because the lettering on the Certificate is different from that in the Act. Thus, in the Act, 1(1)(a) is C or D on Certificate A, (b) is B, (c) is A, (d) is E. This anomaly may be corrected in the near future.

28 General Medical Council (1998) *Good Medical Practice*. GMC, London, para. 14.

29 See the story of Abram and Hagar, Sarah's maid, in *Genesis* 16.

30 DoH (1984) *Report of the Committee of Inquiry into Human Fertilisation and Embryology*. HMSO, London, para. 8.1.

31 Kant I (1991) *Groundwork of the Metaphysic of Morals* translated by Paton HJ. Routledge, London.

32 This is often referred to as 'commodification', a term also applied to the sale of organs.

33 The Surrogacy Arrangements Act 1985 as amended by the Human Fertilisation and Embryology Act 1990 s 30.

CHAPTER EIGHT

Children: 'When will I be old enough?'

Summary

Ethical dilemmas in paediatrics are mainly concerned with consent to treatment. Who is able to give consent, and what governs that ability? Paramount in all decision making is the protection of the interests of the child. The issues are considered as far as possible in chronological order, followed by sections on the law and research in children:

- The developing foetus
- The infant and preschool child
- The schoolchild
- Puberty and adolescence
- Children as research subjects
- The law and children

I remember at that time I went to the hairdressers . . . next to me was a young mother with a little girl aged about three. The child, whose hair was about to be cut for the first time, screamed with terror and clung to her mother. The hairdresser stood by gravely, comb in hand: he recognised that this was a serious moment.[1]

Introduction

In our society, children occupy a special place where they are considered more vulnerable to damage than the rest of the population.

Consequently, those responsible for their care have a legal and ethical duty to protect them, from the moment of birth to adulthood. Indeed, some sections of society consider that this responsibility begins before birth, although in legal terms this does not necessarily apply (*see* also Chapter 7).[2]

In most families, it is the parents who have this specific nurturing responsibility for the child, and the doctor acts as an adjunct. As Lord Templeman said:

> The best person to bring up a child is the natural parent. It matters not whether the parent is wise or foolish, rich or poor, educated or illiterate, provided the child's moral and physical health are not endangered. Public authorities cannot improve on nature.[3]

It is in this age group that children will begin to be self-reliant and able to make decisions for themselves. Information and explanation ought to be given to child and parents together, with the intention that agreement can be reached with all the parties involved: child, parent and doctor. Ignoring the child would be removing any right the child has to decide for himself.

It is only when the parents decide that their sick child requires medical attention that the doctor will be involved. Likewise, medical surveillance of the normal child – developmental checks, immunisations – can only be carried out with the cooperation and consent of the parents.[4]

The growing child will gradually mature from a state of complete dependence as a neonate towards physical and intellectual independence in adolescence. The age at which maturity occurs varies from one individual to another, and even from one situation to another in the same individual; physical maturity may predate intellectual maturity by a number of years. It is important to understand that absolute care and control of the infant will need to be relinquished gradually as the child grows up and becomes the equivalent of an autonomous adult.

This chapter will identify some of the common ethical dilemmas that can occur when treating children. For example, ethical problems will certainly arise in the medical care of children where the parent, the doctor and the child disagree in the decision-making process. The law, as it relates to the medical care of children, will be introduced at relevant points. In our society, the legal protection of a child's interests is well-defined, and usually, but not always, coincides with ethical reasoning.

Increasingly, it is recognised that the child himself can be, and ought to be, involved in decision making. We have already stated that children mature at very different rates; even quite young children can understand the implications of their illness and choices of treatment. This means that ethical decisions ought only to be made after the child has been given the *opportunity* to express his wishes about medical examination, investigation and treatment. He can only do this if a realistic attempt has been made to achieve his understanding. If we ignore this opportunity, the competent child is denied an important right, his autonomy may be compromised, and we are behaving unethically.

It is not difficult to envisage where problems may arise, if we accept this premise. It will take time and commitment on the part of the doctor to find out exactly how much the individual child is *capable* of understanding in order to make an informed choice. The doctor and the parents may already have decided on the best option on behalf of the child, and may have some difficulty in resisting an attempt to influence the child in that direction, particularly where the child is unwilling to 'cooperate'. The particular circumstances are also important: a child may be competent to decide if faced with one situation, and have difficulty comprehending another, at a different time. For example, a sick child may behave in a more mature way when convalescent than when he was acutely ill. Life-threatening conditions produce specific problems if the child is deemed competent yet refuses treatment. In such an extreme situation the court may be asked to intervene.[5]

The developing foetus

The baby, before it is born, has no legal rights. In law, the pregnant mother's rights are legally paramount. This is perhaps the most ethically troubling aspect of antenatal care. The general practitioner will only rarely be faced with this as a problem, for example where the expectant mother is adamant about her plan for confinement and where this plan is in direct conflict with the probability of a safely delivered normal infant. It is worrying enough where the mother's wish will jeopardise her own health, but somehow worse where the baby's life is at risk. Nevertheless, it has proved impossible for the courts to override the woman's decision in favour of the foetus.[6]

The doctor's ethical duty to the mother in such a situation is clear. The woman is entitled to a balanced explanation of all the risks involved, both to her and the child, so that she is in a position to make an informed decision. However strongly the doctor feels about her irrationality, as it might affect the child in the future, her autonomy ought to be respected (*see* Chapter 7). Yet it is understandable that a GP in this situation might also wish to persuade the mother to comply with medical advice, particularly as the foetus matures and term approaches.

This is another example where Foot's mandatory and elective ethical principles are helpful (*see* Chapter 7).[7] Although the mother has a rights claim to have her autonomy respected, the nearly mature child could be regarded as having certain rights in a counter claim. To phrase it more strongly, according to an elective principle, a course of action aimed at saving the child from harm is ethically preferable to a course of action allowing the mother to indulge in her irrational and harmful desire. It is perhaps unfortunate that the law is unsupportive in this respect (*see* Chapter 7).[8]

The infant and preschool child

Quality of parenthood

There are frequent contacts made with the GP by the parents of the under-fives. Apart from developmental checks and immunisations, there will be the need for advice on feeding, sleeping and behavioural problems as well as minor illnesses. These contacts offer the GP the opportunity to observe the development of relationships within the family, attitudes of the parents towards their children, and parental competence. It will only be when something seems to be going wrong that the GP will be inclined to intervene.

> Adam was born 2 days ago to Barbara after a normal first pregnancy and confinement. The GP is visiting mother and baby at home, when Barbara asks the GP to arrange for Adam's circumcision. She says that she is not very keen on the idea, but there is strong pressure from her in-laws, as 'all the men were done as babies'.

Is this a reasonable and straightforward request? Barbara has expressed her opinion, if rather diffidently. The GP does not know yet what her husband has to say, but his parents are very clear on 'the family norm'. Adam, as a neonate, has his decisions made for him by his parents, but may have a very definite opinion later in life. There are different views of the surgery involved, from one extreme – a painful mutilation – to the other – a painless improvement on nature. The GP will have a view, influenced as much by his culture as his medical experience.

Consider the ethical principle *'primum non nocere'* – above all, do no harm. Gillon calls this a 'shibboleth' of traditional medical ethics, arguing that such a principle, which insists on the priority of non-maleficence over all other ethical considerations, is particularly unhelpful.[9] We could say that circumcision would harm Adam, and it would be wrong to agree to a referral. Alternatively we could say that there ought to be a referral: Barbara's unwillingness as a parent to agree to pressure from the baby's paternal relatives ought to be overridden in the interests of future benign relationships within the family – thus preventing harm in that important area.

It is impossible to predict such an outcome without knowing Adam's father's view. He may be doubtful, like his wife, but have difficulty in confronting his parents and their strong views. The GP's advice and support could be very helpful to him. He is the father in his own little family now, and may need to develop that role independently from his own parents. If, however, he is as keen on Adam's circumcision as his parents, and the GP is unhappy to refer, what is then the *duty* of the GP? As we shall see later in this chapter, there would be no *legal* sanction against this procedure.

The ethical complexity of what seemed at first to be a simple and straightforward request from Barbara is becoming apparent. It would be easy – and legally safe – to comply with such a request, and many GPs would do so.[10] Yet some GPs would be very concerned about recommending the procedure, which is not without distress and risk to the baby. A doctor with a 'conscientious objection' to a procedure is on the one hand released from the duty of acting personally, but is obliged to fulfil another duty, that of informing the patient how they can get help elsewhere (*see* Chapter 7, section on abortion).[11] In discussing the issue with Adam's parents, the GP will need to be very clear in his own mind that his concerns are well-founded on Adam's best interests, and are not grounded in his own prejudices or beliefs.

Congenital abnormalities

Parents hope for a normal baby to be born to them. When this does not happen, and the baby that arrives is not perfect, they are likely to be distraught, and enter a bereavement process for the normal baby that never came. After the initial shock at birth or neonatal diagnosis, caring for a child with significant abnormalities puts a great strain on the family; the GP will recognise how important it is to provide as much support as is possible within the practice team.

Every GP will have a family on his list which includes a child with Down's syndrome. A recent survey by the UK Down's Syndrome Association suggests that these children are not getting the same level of medical care that is provided for normal children. The fact that they have Down's syndrome can adversely affect the treatment decisions made by doctors.[12] We know that sometimes parents and doctors are faced with very difficult ethical decisions regarding the treatment of critically ill neonates. In general practice it is the ongoing everyday care which is criticised. If the criticism is valid, is it possible morally to rebut it?

Consent to treatment: implied

It is assumed when a small child is brought by its parent to see the doctor that implicit consent has been given to examination and treatment by the very fact that the child is presented to the GP with that in mind. This is the same assumption made when treating competent adults (*see* Chapter 2).

Nevertheless, it is important to make sure that the parent understands the reasons for any examination or procedure that affects their child. Likewise, the GP will need to understand the parent's concerns. Parents sometimes have to make some difficult choices on behalf of their children; it is the GP's moral duty to inform, explain and support them at these times.

Immunisations

In the case of immunisations, it is usual practice to seek *formal* consent and a parent's signature to confirm consent is required. Parents are naturally anxious about the possible dangers of vaccines, an anxiety fuelled by media reports of vaccine-damaged children. They may be confused when faced with what they perceive as a choice between protection of their baby against an infectious disease, the incidence of which is very low, and the possibility of actively inflicting harm on the child through vaccine damage. In mathematical terms, the relative risk of vaccine side-effects will rise as the risk of acquiring a disease is reduced.

This issue is becoming more difficult now that the incidence of serious infectious disease in childhood has been reduced dramatically, and is outside the experience of most young parents. The statement that the introduction and widespread use of vaccination has made the biggest contribution to this reduction may not impress some parents, even though their babies now are benefiting from actions taken by parents in the past. They may say that the incidence of these diseases was already declining when vaccination programmes were introduced, and this decline could be attributed to a better standard of living and improvement in public health generally.[13]

The controversy over the safety of the combined measles/mumps/rubella (MMR) vaccine was started by an article in the medical press which was widely reported in the media at the time.[14] As a result many parents refused to have their children immunised, and the anxiety persists in some in spite of subsequent rejection of the researchers' findings by further research and the Chief Medical Officers for England and Wales.[15]

We could question the moral rectitude of the manner in which the media report medical matters, which is a much wider reportage than childhood immunisation. Once the public, or a group of people such as parents of young children, have absorbed one side of an argument and formed an opinion, it is exceedingly difficult to change that opinion to a more balanced one. Research by Leask and Chapman has shown that reports in the media claiming that vaccines are dangerous and ineffective are attached in the mind of the public to fears of commercial and government conspiracy and cover up. Such fears are difficult to dislodge. Is the damage done by such a slant outweighed by the social benefit? Or, as Leask and Chapman state, 'what we have learned from immunisation science will be of no public value ultimately if we ignore key lessons from health communication science.'[16]

This is an example where immunisation of the older infant not only protects that child against disease but also, by reducing the incidence in the population, reduces the risk dramatically for the younger more vulnerable baby. The GP is well aware of the arguments supporting vaccination. For example, in areas where the uptake of MMR vaccination has fallen, the incidence of measles is beginning to increase. Where measles has become a rare disease, it is easy to forget its serious and life-threatening complications. Like measles, mumps is not always a benign illness. The rubella vaccination programme has meant that the possibility of rubella damage to the foetus, a valid reason for termination of pregnancy, is now uncommon.

Clare has come to see the GP for a routine pill check. The health visitor has alerted the GP to the fact that Clare's son Danny is overdue for his MMR. The GP suggests to Clare that she brings him to the clinic for this to be done. It is especially important, as the GP has just seen the first two cases of measles in the area for a long time. She responds firmly, that in no way is Danny going to get the MMR vaccination. Her neighbour's young son is autistic and she does not want Danny to be subjected to anything that might put him at risk – she knows what autism means to a family.

There are important and conflicting ethical issues that arise in this initially straightforward consultation:

- the duty of the mother to protect her child and the rest of the family from harm
- the duty of the GP to protect the health of the child – beneficence
- the duty of the GP not to harm the child – non-maleficence

balanced against

- the future benefit to the health of the community – utility

balanced against

- the right of a mother to decide for her child.

Where does the doctor's duty lie? The aim of the utilitarian might be satisfied by the right of the community to a vaccination programme that protected *all* children, even if there was a risk to a minority. As defined by JJC Smart, 'act-utilitarianism is the view that the rightness or wrongness of an action is to be judged by the consequences, good or bad, of the action itself.'[17]

A balance needs to be struck between the degree of protection to the majority and the quantified risk to the minority. As Smart goes on to say in making his distinction between act- and rule-utilitarianism: 'rule-utilitarianism is the view that the rightness or wrongness of an action is to be judged by the goodness or badness of the consequences of a rule that everyone should perform the action in like circumstances.'[17] Under this 'rule', in terms of overall benefit to humanity, there could be an argument for a coercive, or even compulsory, approach.[18] Doctors are in a position to *persuade* parents to submit their children to vaccination, as a recommended treatment, even if the parents feel it is not in their *individual* child's best interests to comply. It is possible to give more emphasis to the vaccine's safety and benefits than its risks in the information offered to parents; if research evidence is flimsy, but is exaggerated by the media, doctors could feel justified in discounting evidence of risk to their patients. It remains in doubt whether this approach is morally sound.

Parents are likely to see their duty to their own child of paramount importance. They could have some difficulty in being altruistic in considering the good of others even when they know that the risk to their child is tiny – *no* risk is acceptable to them. If the utilitarian principle is rejected, the moral demand on the doctor is then to consider what is best for each individual child in the family context. This deontological view is based on the autonomy of the family unit. It will conflict with the utilitarian view, particularly if future research evidence confirms a measurable risk of vaccine damage to some children.

> Bearing these arguments in mind, what do you say to Clare?

The screaming toddler and the room-wrecker

The management of a consultation with a screaming, uncooperative child patient, or a child who roams around the room incessantly, opening drawers and cupboards and behaving destructively, is not easy. It is a familiar scenario to most GPs, and each will deal with it in his or her own way.

The ethical dimension is not apparent at first. The child's parent has had enough concern to bring the child to the surgery, and has some expectations of the doctor. Unless the prime reason for attendance is behavioural, the parent will be either apologetic or oblivious of any problem.

These are children who are refusing intervention, and whose behaviour has the potential of distracting the GP from the task. Of the choices of negotiation, coercion, bribery and physical force, only the first has ethical credibility – and is the one least likely to be successful in the very young child.

It is important to remember that a doctor can only work within the limits set by the patient, or in this case, the parent and child. The parent is consenting on behalf of the child, yet the child is strongly resisting attempts at clinical examination. The GP has a contractual duty to the patient, as well as a moral duty to promote the patient's good (beneficence rather than non-maleficence).

> How far ought the doctor to pursue a clinical examination in the face of a small child's opposition?

The schoolchild

Parental control

It is in this age group that children will begin to be self-reliant and able to make decisions for themselves. Information and explanation ought to be given to the child and parents together with the intention that agreement can be reached with all the parties involved: child, parent and doctor. Ignoring the child would be removing any right the child has to decide for himself.

Conflicts begin to arise as the child matures and becomes more understanding of the implications of health and disease. Parental concern over some aspect of health or symptom expressed by the child will bring them to see the GP, but as with the younger patient, the older child may be resistant to control by the parent. The GP has to steer a course between the two of them, parent and child, which is ultimately beneficial to the child as well as fostering compliance.

Sharing concerns with others

The GP, like the health visitor and the school nurse, is in a prime position to discover the first signs of child abuse, physical or sexual. Awareness of a link between a symptom or sign and child abuse tends to be subliminal unless the child is already known to be in a high-risk family. Once there is a suspicion in the mind of the GP it is often quite difficult to know how to deal with it. Obviously, in a clear cut emergency situation there are important contacts to be made immediately; but if there is only a very slight suspicion, is there going to be more harm brought about to the child and the family by notifying another body? Where does the greater risk lie?

Very bad news

As with adults, sometimes the GP can be faced with a sick child presenting with strong evidence of a serious disease, perhaps a malignancy. This situation requires great sensitivity, particularly as the child's parents' understanding and fears of 'the worst' may already have been transmitted to the child. It is not always easy to assess how much of an explanation the child will be able to understand. Treating the child patient at a level too far below the child's level of intellectual comprehension would be wrong, just as the reverse – expectations pitched too high for the child – would be wrong as well.

Ellie is 8 years old. She has not been well for a few weeks, nothing specific, a few fevers and loss of appetite. She went out to a friend's birthday treat today, but had to be brought home early because she was too tired to walk and had to be pushed in a push chair. The same evening her mother Frances brings her to see the GP as an emergency. On history and examination, the most likely diagnosis is leukaemia until proved otherwise. The GP advises immediate hospital admission to the local children's cancer unit.

Unless the child is deliberately excluded from the room, he or she will be privy to any discussion that takes place between the GP and the parent. The words that the GP uses to inform the parent will usually be understood by the child. As will happen in this case, the GP will need to arrange an admission over the telephone, explaining the reason clearly to the hospital doctor. Medical euphemisms may convey enough information but do not always disguise a sense of urgency. If the GP is too anxious in attempting to minimise distress in both parent and child, the reality may be too heavily submerged. This results in false reassurance for the family. Will they be able to trust a doctor to tell them the truth in future?

How ought the consultation with Ellie and her mother to be handled by the GP?

Puberty and adolescence

There are some ethical issues that are more specific to this group of children. As puberty approaches, the child's autonomy begins to develop. Through adolescence the parent's authority diminishes and the child becomes self-reliant and competent to make important decisions on his or her own account. This growing up process can be quite challenging for parents especially when their child gets into difficulties.

The list of possible areas of ethical conflict is substantial:

- compliance/rebellion and the silent or monosyllabic patient
- protecting confidentiality, especially from parents
- the unaccompanied child – Gillick competence and consent to treatment
- pregnancy
- substance abuse
- eating disorders
- depression
- irrational beliefs
- refusing treatment
- the parent as proxy for the absent child patient.

Some of these are closely connected with each other: it would be unhelpful and tedious to consider each in isolation. The overall picture will emerge of a group of individuals who are testing out the adult world, each in his or her own way but with one attribute in common: that of the willingness if not the capacity to learn from new experiences. Unfortunately, the young person's behaviour can be inexplicable and worrying for the parents, who may expect the GP to produce an acceptable answer to their problems.

When concerned parents try to place their burden onto the shoulders of the GP, inevitably the GP risks being drawn into a paternalistic role thus denying the existence of a developing autonomy in the adolescent. This particular attitude is voiced by Foreman who states that 'adolescents lack the social independence needed to make fully autonomous decisions, being vulnerable to external pressures, and benefiting from firm guidance.'[19] It is this firm guidance which the parent wishes the GP to provide, and which the older child may resent most strongly.

George has started to get mild acne. His mother Helen knows that this can be treated. With this in mind she takes him to see the GP. It is Helen who gives the story to the GP and who answers the GP's questions. George is silent, but his facial expression and posture show a distinctly hostile attitude to both adults. Direct questions to him from the GP reveal that he does not accept that he has a problem and he does not want any treatment.

Differences of opinion between parent and child are frequent. In this case, the disagreement does not seem very important: George has spots. He says he can tolerate them but his mother cannot. She may have other concerns, but today, this is the presenting problem for the GP to deal with. It is probably immaterial in terms of harm to George whether he is given a prescription today or not – the condition is not life-threatening. It may, however, be quite important for the family that the GP recognises the conflict between George's growing autonomy and his mother's diminishing power to act as proxy for her son.

What are the ethical arguments that George's GP might use in a decision whether or not to prescribe?

The unaccompanied child

It is usually inadvisable for a GP to see a child under the age of 16 on their own unless they have a responsible adult with them, who is normally a parent or older sibling. The adult need not be present throughout the consultation: often it is very helpful to see the child on his own with the adult waiting outside. The reason for this rule is that in law, a child under the age of 16 is not considered competent to consent to or refuse medical examination or treatment. There are of course important exceptions to this rule that will be discussed more fully later in this chapter.

How does this rule work in practice? Should the GP's staff be instructed to turn away all underage children unless they have a parent or parent's deputy with them? How much of a disadvantage is this to the competent autonomous 15-year-old needing the help and support that can be provided by the GP?

> Ian has just had sex for the first time with his girlfriend Jenny. He did not use a condom. He is worried on two counts: first, about the spots on his scrotum he has noticed since then, and secondly, that he has made her pregnant. They come to see Ian's GP together. They are both 15 years old. Jenny is registered elsewhere.

A consultation such as this exemplifies typical problems that young people bring to a GP that they trust. They rely on the GP to give them sound advice, to treat them in a straightforward manner and perhaps most of all to respect their confidence. It is unlikely that their parents have been told of the plan to visit the GP, or if they have been told, the real reason for the visit would have been kept from them.

The GP who is confronted by these two young people will need to consider the ethical and legal components of the consultation as well as the clinical problems. They have come as a couple: Jenny is an integral part of the interaction although she has a different GP. They are both 'underage' – the legal implications of this are discussed later in this chapter. If they are 'Gillick competent' – and their appearance together in the surgery today seeking help goes a considerable way towards confirming that they are – the GP has a clear duty to respond as best he can to their concerns. His duty will extend towards the reassurance that their confidence will be protected.

However, there is a dilemma if the GP discovers that either one of them is at serious risk – perhaps of sexually transmitted disease, perhaps of pregnancy. This is particularly concerning if it becomes clear on questioning that they are adamant that they will not involve their parents, nor is the GP to do so. In this situation, the *legal* principle becomes important in upholding the *ethical* management – that of proper *clinical* treatment. If Gillick competence is proven by the GP, treatment must be given; if it is not, an adult with parental responsibility must be involved.

The parent as proxy for the child patient

Sometimes a worried parent will consult the GP in the absence of the child. The parent has noticed something untoward in the child's behaviour, or maybe the school has initiated the contact because the teachers have become concerned. The main fears seem to be of substance abuse or an eating disorder, but there may be others. Without the actual patient being present any discussion will be founded on conjecture.

A comparison can be drawn with the absent adult patient; an example would be that of a husband who gives to their GP a clear story of alcohol dependence in his wife. The GP can offer support to the husband but inevitably this will fall short of dealing with the wife's problem unless she attends in person.

However, there is a fundamental difference between the adult and the child. The adult's responsibility to his wife, another adult, does not extend to the ability and requirement to make decisions on her behalf. The responsibilities of a parent towards his child were described at the beginning of this chapter, and are based on the need to protect the vulnerable child from harm until that child reaches maturity.

The practical difficulty remains: the GP cannot begin to resolve the parent's anxiety without seeing the child, both with the parent present and with the child alone. Once the child is there, a further ethical dilemma presents itself, a dilemma not made any easier by the law. How far ought the GP to protect the confidentiality of a child?

Kate's mother Laura has been to see the GP because she and Kate's teachers are worried about her. Until the last few months Kate was an active lively girl, accomplished at sport and in her school work. Of late she has become preoccupied, withdrawn, eats very little and is disinterested in friends and hobbies, although her school work is not suffering. At home she spends all her time in her room and does not communicate with her parents. Laura is even more concerned as she has found books on pagan rituals hidden in Kate's room: Laura herself has a strong religious faith.

If Kate is persuaded to see the GP and does so on her own, and if she expects secrecy, she may feel encouraged to divulge confidential information that may put the GP in a difficult position. How far ought Kate's confidence to be protected? Laura will be interested to know what her daughter has told the GP. The GP may have made a clinical diagnosis of depression: counselling and medication will be options. Kate's competence to consent to treatment will depend on whether she is 'Gillick competent'(*see* below). The question here is rather different: is she competent *also* to understand all the implications of secrecy and expectations of confidence?

Children as research subjects

Although GPs occasionally take part in research projects involving their adult patients, the use of children as research subjects is not a topic relevant to primary care. It is relevant, however, to consider the treatments that a GP will prescribe for his child patients and how, or even whether, they have achieved a product licence for use in children. Also, all children who are entered into hospital-based research trials will be registered with a GP. If such trials do not take place, potentially useful drugs will not get a licence for use in children; if they are used, this will be unlicensed, or 'off-label', rendering the prescriber vulnerable to legal action if damage due to the drug is proven.

There are three main areas of ethical concern:

- consent – how far is the child included in the process?
- altruism or coercion – how is consent governed?
- good of others – how does this balance with an estimate of any harm to child?

The British Paediatric Association (BPA) has produced guidelines on research in children. The document makes some important points.

1   Research in children is important and should be supported.
2   Children have unique interests and are not mini-adults.
3   Research is only ethical in children if it cannot be done in adults equally well.

4 The child's agreement must be secured.
5 Any procedure not directly benefiting the child should satisfy legal and ethical principles of minimal risk.[20]

The law and children

We will find that the law protects the interests of children in a way that coincides admirably with the ethical principles of beneficence, non-maleficence and justice, and now, following the Gillick case,[21] with the acknowledgement of a child's progress towards autonomy.

The child's interests are governed by the following statutes and common law:

• Family Law Reform Act 1969
• Children Act 1989
• the Gillick case.

Best interests

This is a phrase which is frequently used when difficult decisions need to be made involving those patients who are not able to give full informed consent to a procedure, and where consent is required from another acting as legal proxy: either an individual or an authority.[22] It is important to clarify exactly what we mean by this in each individual case. The law provides us with a *minimal* standard of behaviour. It is interesting to note that the law inclines to the view that an 'invasive medical procedure' can still be in the patient's best interests even if it is not medically needed, carries with it some risks, or even if it is primarily to be performed in the interests of a third party.

Baby Adam's circumcision,[23] according to case law, could therefore be perfectly legal.[24] As Munby points out, 'ritual or other non-therapeutic circumcision of minor male children is ... permissible ...' If we agree that medical ethics demands of us rather more than the law, that we are looking for *optimum* standards of behaviour, the decision to refer Adam for circumcision for a non-medical reason becomes more of a problem. It is the consideration of the *ethical* rather than the *legal* implications that may cause concern to his GP.

Nonetheless, we need to be able to make an attempt at defining more clearly in ethical terms what is meant by the phrase 'best interests'. Perhaps it is helpful if we return to the basic ethical principles originally outlined in the Hippocratic Oath (*see* Appendix 1). The main principle will be to act in a way that promotes the child's health and welfare and avoid any action that might be harmful to the child. Although a second principle would uphold the right of a competent child to exercise autonomy in decisions, the right of that child to refuse life-saving treatment would collide with the preservation of the child's best interests as defined. In law, the child's refusal is most likely to be overridden, if not by the parents, then by the courts. For example, a child needing a life-saving blood tranfusion may be judged competent to consent to the procedure; if the child refuses, perhaps because of firmly held religious beliefs which may be shared by the parents, the court can override the refusal and sanction the transfusion.[25]

This level of ethical conflict is unlikely to impinge on everyday general practice. Nonetheless, it is important to be aware that such conflicts exist together with the question of what truly constitutes a child's best interests. In many cases, upholding a child's decision against that of the parents may be in the child's best interests.

> Ian's girlfriend Jenny finds she is pregnant. She wishes to continue the pregnancy but her parents, in particular her father, are insisting that she has a termination. They take her along to the family's GP saying that he must arrange for this as soon as possible. They are not prepared to support her and the child, nor will they allow her to interrupt her education.

In law, Jenny may be competent to consent to treatment. If she consults her GP wishing to be referred for termination and she is judged competent, then it is lawful for her to consent, even if she is under 16 years of age. Can she refuse an abortion in the face of her parents' opposition to her decision to proceed with the pregnancy?

In resolving this deadlock, given that the criteria of the Abortion Act are satisfied in her case, yet her family has threatened to withdraw support for her and her child, it is necessary to refer to the definition of 'best interests'.

> What action by the GP furthers Jenny's best interests?

The Family Law Reform Act 1969

Using the curious terminology of legal documents this statute refers to those under the age of 18 as 'infants'. Yet, in law, those over the age of 16 may consent to 'medical, surgical or dental treatment' which will include diagnostic and other associated procedures. Between the ages of 16 and 18 the law appears to be interested only in refusals of treatment that are against the child's best interests.[26] It is in this age group that the court can continue to overrule a young person's refusal until at the age of 18 when the child automatically becomes *sui juris*: of full age and therefore independent. Under the age of 16 a child is deemed incompetent to consent unless 'Gillick competence' can be demonstrated (*see* below).

Children Act 1989

This statute provides for guardianship, or parental responsibility, for children. Where medical treatment is concerned, the Act dictates who can act as proxy for a child and consent to treatment. It will normally be the parent, but if there is a conflict between parents and doctors, doctors can apply to the court for approval for treatment or for withholding of treatment if the parents' decision appears to be against child's best interests: the court can concur with or override decisions by parents or guardians in order to uphold the child's best interests. The court is said to be exercising its *inherent parens patriae jurisdiction*.[27] There is, of course, no guarantee that the court will uphold the doctors who wish to override the parents; if it does not, the court in its wisdom will appear to have infringed the doctors' discretion. The other main cause for the court to be involved is for consent to organ donation. The court is the only body that can consent to this on behalf of a minor, until the child has reached the age of 18. The only other time that a child who is not yet Gillick competent (*see* below) can be treated without the parent's consent is in an emergency, either when the parent is not available, or when the parent has withheld consent against the child's best interests.

Gillick competence: the concept of the mature minor

The case that brought the phrase 'Gillick competence' into being was brought by Mrs Gillick. It had a protracted course through the courts and eventually ended up in the House of Lords. The judgement and subsequent interpretation is crucial to the treatment of children under the age of 16 by GPs. Until that time, a GP who was consulted by such a child was legally bound to obtain consent from the child's parents before any examination or treatment took place under the provisions of Section 8 of the Family Reform Act 1969. If he did not abide by this he could be prosecuted by the parents. In spite of this, many GPs felt that it was in a child's best interests to ignore this possibility where the child was already sexually active and ran a very real risk of becoming pregnant. If the doctor could argue that the child's best interests overrode parental refusal of consent, then a successful prosecution would be unlikely.

Mrs Gillick was the mother of a large family with several daughters. She was concerned that her daughters would be given contraceptive advice or prescribed the contraceptive pill without her knowledge and consent; she considered that it was for the parent, not the doctor, to judge what was in the best interests of the child. Her action was based on this view and she wished the courts to endorse it and to support the power of veto by parents on treatment of their children. In her view, it was wrong for doctors to give contraceptive advice to children as this would encourage sexual activity in the young person that was not in the child's best interests. In medical terms, it could be said that early sexual activity is associated with certain health risks: apart from the obvious one of unwanted pregnancy, there would be possible exposure to sexually transmitted disease (STD) such as chlamydia and human papilloma virus. In view of this how morally persuasive is Mrs Gillick's argument?

On the other hand, prior to 1986, GPs already had the experience of consultations with young people who were sexually active, with little intention of stopping, and who could benefit from sensible advice on sexual activities and relationships as well as on contraception. Prevention of pregnancy and STDs in this age group, without the necessity of parental intervention, was deemed to be of paramount importance. Many of these patients would have been inhibited from seeing the GP if they knew that the GP would inform their parents. The GP could argue that treating these patients without their parents' knowledge was a damage limitation exercise entailing more beneficence that harm. How morally persuasive is this argument in contrast to that of Mrs Gillick?

Having described the background to the Gillick case we turn to its significance. Since 1986 the law has recognised the gradual maturation of a child that reaches an adult level of competence in stages unrelated to chronological age. Different children will reach this level at different ages, but once they are competent, parental authority can no longer be applied. As Lord Scarman said at the appeal: 'I would hold that as a matter of law the parental right to determine whether or not their minor child below the age of 16 will have medical treatment terminates if and when that child achieves a sufficient understanding and intelligence to enable him or her to understand fully what is proposed.' He went further in referring to *fact*: 'It will be a question of fact whether a child seeking advice has sufficient understanding of what is involved to give a consent valid in law ...'[28] It is important to note that there is no discrimination between the sexes; although Mrs Gillick brought her action on behalf of her daughters, the judgement covers both boys and girls.

The term 'Gillick competent' has come to be used to describe a child who has reached a stage of intellectual maturity enough to be able to consent to proposed treatment, as described by Lord Scarman. The child who is able to:

- understand the medical advice
- understand the nature, implications and consequences of the proposed treatment together with any risks
- understand the family and moral implications of treatment

will be deemed to have the capacity to consent.[29] As a result of this case, GPs are reassured that the law allows them to treat a child under 16 in the child's best interests without informing the parents providing the child is Gillick competent. It is expected that the child will be encouraged by the GP to inform his or her parents but there is no legal obligation to go beyond this.[30]

Confidentiality

The GP is also protecting the child's confidentiality, an obligation that is endorsed by the Gillick judgement. The same criteria apply: in order to be competent to have his or her confidence protected the child will need to understand what an obligation of confidence entails.[31] Of course there would be the exception that if the competent child wished to pursue a course which was clearly *against* his best interests, such as refusing vital treatment, the doctor could break confidence in the public interest and notify the child's parents. If child abuse or criminal activity by the parents was disclosed by the child, others apart from the parents will need to be involved by the GP.

The ethical principle of respect for autonomy underlies the recognition of Gillick competence in a minor and has been endorsed by the courts. It is for the GP to make a well-reasoned judgement of a child patient's competence, both for consent to treatment and the obligation of confidentiality, in order to treat the child in an ethical way.

Conclusion

It is important to remember that the ethical consideration of the treatment of children evolves as the child develops from a dependent infant to a fully autonomous adult. Each child needs individual consideration at each stage and for each medical issue that arises. It is important to remember that children must be treated as equal individuals and allowed to influence decisions on their future depending on their maturity.

References and notes

1 Brookner A (1990) *Brief Lives*. Jonathan Cape, London.
2 In a case where a husband wished to prevent his wife having an abortion, the judge Sir George Baker P said 'the foetus cannot, in English law, in my view, have any right of its own at least until it is born.' Paton v Trustees of BPAS (1979) *QB*: 276.

   A working paper produced by the Law Commission in 1973 accepted that in order to have the right the foetus must be born. Yet the civil law does protect the rights of an unborn child where its interests require it. *See* In: Whitfield A (1998). In I Kennedy and A Grubb (eds) *Principles of Medical Law*. Oxford University Press, Oxford, p. 653.
3 Re KD (a minor) (ward: termination of access) (1988) *AC*: 806, 812.
4 This applies in the UK. In the US, however, some childhood immunisations are compulsory.
5 In the commentary by Andrew Grubb on Re C (detention: medical treatment) (1997) **2** *FLR*, where a 16-year-old girl was refusing treatment for anorexia nervosa, it is stated that 'Wall J had no difficulty in determining that a judge of the Family Division exercising the court's inherent jurisdiction could, in principle, override a competent child's refusal of medical treatment and, further, could authorise the use of reasonable force to effect that treatment.' *Medical Law Review* (1997) p. 231.
6 In Re MB (1997) **2** *FLR*, where a woman refused caesarian section for malpresentation, Butler-Sloss LJ said that 'a competent woman may... choose not to have medical intervention even though... the consequence may be the death or serious handicap of the child she bears...'
7 Freeman M (1998) Medically Assisted Reproduction. In: I Kennedy and A Grubb (eds) *Principles of Medical Law*. Oxford University Press, Oxford, p. 569.
8 St George's Healthcare NHS Trust v S, R v Collins and others, ex parte (1998) **3** *All ER*: 673.
9 Gillon R (1995) *Philosophical Medical Ethics*. Wiley, Chichester, Ch. 13.
10 The GP may be influenced by a paper indicating that male circumcision gives some protection against HIV infection and 'should be seriously considered as an additional means of preventing HIV in all countries with a high prevalence of infection'. Szabo R and Short RV (2000) How does male circumcision protect against HIV infection? *BMJ*. **320**: 1592–4.
11 General Medical Council (1998) *Good Medical Practice*. GMC, London, p. 6, 'If you feel that your beliefs might affect the treatment you provide, you must explain this to patients, and tell them of their right to see another doctor.'
12 Mayor S (1999) Parents of people with Down's syndrome report suboptimal care. *BMJ*. **318**: 687.

13 Bedford H and Elliman D (2000) Concerns about immunisation. *BMJ*. **320**: 240–3.

14 Wakefield AJ, Murch SH, Linnell AAJ *et al.* (1998) Ileal-lymphoid-nodular hyperplasia, non-specific colitis and pervasive developmental disorder in children. *Lancet*. **351**: 637–41.

15 An information leaflet for parents quotes a personal message from Professor Sir Kenneth Calman acknowledging that 'the decision to immunise your child is never simple'. Calman K (1998) *MMR – the facts*. Health Education Authority, London.

16 Leask JA, Chapman S and Hawe P (2000) Facts are not enough. *BMJ*. **321**: 108–9 (letter).

17 Smart JJC (1973) An outline of a system of utilitarian ethics. In: *Utilitarianism – for and against*. Cambridge University Press, Cambridge.

18 A recent unsubstantiated rumour in the United States was reported by some parents. This was a threat to remove children from the custody of their parents if they failed to receive a recommended vaccine. *Letter from Dr JM Orient, Medical Director, Association of American Physicians and Surgeons, to Dr SL Katz*, 25 October 1999.

19 Foreman DM (1999) The family rule: a framework for obtaining ethical consent for medical intervention from children. *J Med Ethics*. **25**(6): 491–6.

20 Ethics Advisory Committee BPA (1992) *Guidelines for the Ethical Conduct of Medical Research Involving Children*. British Paediatric Association, London.

21 Gillick v West Norfolk and Wisbech Area Health Authority (1986) *AC*: 112.

22 Munby J (1998) Consent to treatment: children and the incompetent patient. In: I Kennedy and A Grubb (eds) *Principles of Medical Law*. Oxford University Press, Oxford, p. 247.

23 *Ibid.* p. 247, footnote 387. 'Circumcision is normally of no medical benefit and devoid of rational justification . . . is not without risks and . . . can lead to complications, serious injury, and even death.'

24 Re F (mental patient: sterilisation) (1990) **2** *AC*: 1. This case is important in that it uses the principle of necessity as the basis of the judgement, to allow the non-therapeutic sterilisation of an incompetent adult, in that person's 'best interests'.

25 Re R (a minor) (blood transfusion) (1993) **2** *FLR*.

26 Consent between the ages of 16 and 18 is covered by Section 8 of the Family Law Reform Act 1969 and does not include organ donation or, indeed, donation of blood or blood products such as marrow. Defining the child's best interests will govern proxy consent in this age group as with the young child.

27 Facility for the court to take parental responsibility without necessarily making the child a ward of court.

28   Gillick v West Norfolk and Wisbech Area Health Authority (1986) *AC*: 112, 188–9.

29   It is interesting to note that the criteria of competence in a child are considerably more stringent than those applied for an adult.

30   There is a useful discussion of the case by Margaret Brazier who quotes Lord Fraser who set out five matters the doctor should satisfy himself on before giving contraceptive treatment to a girl below 16 without parental agreement. They are:

1   that the girl will understand his advice
2   that he cannot persuade her to inform her parents
3   that she is very likely to begin or continue having sexual intercourse with or without contraceptive treatment
4   that unless she receives contraceptive advice or treatment her physical or mental health or both are likely to suffer
5   that her best interests require him to give her contraceptive advice or treatment or both without the parental consent.

But she reminds us that doctors are not yet free from the threat of legal action by angry parents discovering that their child has been given contraception. As Lord Scarman said, 'Clearly a doctor who gives a brief contraceptive advice or treatment not because in his clinical judgement the treatment is medically indicated . . . but with the intention of facilitating her having unlawful sexual intercourse may well be guilty of a criminal offence.' The counter-argument would be that the doctor is not encouraging the continuance of sexual intercourse and implicitly the crime of unlawful sexual intercourse, but offering '. . . a palliative against the consequences of crime'.

Brazier M (1992) *Medicine Patients and the Law.* Penguin, Harmondsworth, pp. 336–9.

31   Stern K (1998) Confidentiality and medical records. In: I Kennedy and A Grubb (eds) *Principles of Medical Law.* Oxford University Press, Oxford, pp. 508–9.

CHAPTER NINE

A good death: ethics and humanity at the end of life

Summary

It is a doctor's duty to prolong life, but also to make the process of dying easier. The conflicts that arise between these two aims need careful thought and, if possible, resolution.

- Differences between acts and omissions at the end of life
- Doctrine of Double Effect
- Ordinary and extraordinary treatments
- Futility
- What is euthanasia?
- Legal aspects of euthanasia
- Is there a right to die?
- Advance statements
- Best interests.

... since consciousness is a dynamic condition (that is, you have to choose whether to act or not to act upon your knowledge, and even a decision to remain inactive is an action) it becomes the privilege, not to say duty of conscious beings to move, possibly alter the flow of their times.[1]

Introduction

This chapter will examine the issues surrounding GPs' involvement in the care of dying patients, with attention to the moral problems that this area highlights. Recent years have seen a greater awareness of subjects such as euthanasia, a right to die and advance statements on treatment. In describing these subjects many other ethical issues surface. Medical involvement in the process of dying will be addressed, rather than an analysis of what death means.[2]

First, here are some examples from clinical practice to set the scene.

Arnold is 90 and lives in a residential home for the elderly mentally infirm, due to advanced cerebrovascular dementia. He has little cognitive function and is doubly incontinent. He requires help with feeding and other activities of daily living. Lately he has shown little interest at all in the home activities. His GP visits the home weekly to see the residents, and when asked to do by the care staff. Today he has been called because Arnold is obviously unwell, with a fever and a cough, and he is not drinking or eating. He arranges supportive care only.

Beryl has been suffering from metastatic cancer for about six months, and slowly deteriorating. She lives with her son, who cares for her dutifully and well. She is virtually pain-free, on a drug cocktail. Her other bodily needs are well managed by her family, a palliative care team who visit regularly, and community nursing staff. Of late she has been confined to bed, and needed occasional extra doses of opiate analgesia to remove breakthrough pain. Her GP is visiting one day and is about to administer such a dose. Beryl takes her hand and asks if she would 'release me from all this, when the time comes'. The doctor understands that the meaning of the request is a request for a lethal injection. She is inclined to accept.

Acts and omissions

It is a long-standing principle of ethics that a doctor's decision in situations such as those involving Arnold and Beryl may be deemed morally permissible, or not, on the basis of whether an action or an omission (a failure to act) has brought about an outcome. It could be argued that an omission with subsequent damage attributable to the omission can be morally acceptable, whereas an action giving rise to such damage is not. This assumption needs further analysis.

If her GP accedes to Beryl's request, she performs an action – an injection of a lethal drug. If Arnold is not actively treated, it can be described as an omission – the failure to prescribe a treatment which may save his life. The end, however, may be the same: both patients die. So why are the two situations morally different?

Many philosophers would argue powerfully that they are not different in any sense for the following reasons.

1 Neither GP, if they are honest with themselves, expects the patient to survive. Each of the possible decisions, that of withholding the antibiotic from Arnold and that of injecting Beryl with a lethal dose, could be argued as setting in train a clearly *foreseeable* event – the death of the patient. Both doctors would be choosing to relieve suffering as a treatment aim; this is representative of their duties to their patients.

2 As mentioned above, the *outcome* is the same (or rather might be, as envisioned). Because of this, there is no different moral value attaching to each scenario. This is clearly a consequentialist view: that such value is determined by references to outcome.

3 We might *redefine* the 'inaction' in failing to give Arnold an antibiotic, as an 'action' as follows. At that visit, the GP formed the view that the best treatment for Arnold was to call for further care from the community staff, arranging suitable supportive therapy: attention to hydration and relief of fever, among other things. In essence, this is to select other treatments for the patient, in his best interests. Equally, we could *redefine* the 'action': in following Beryl's request for death as an inaction, Beryl's GP *omitted* to ignore the request. Or, having carried out Beryl's request with, for example, intravenous potassium, she stood by and took no resuscitative measures.

4 To an outside observer what differentiates the two GPs' behaviour is merely a *physical activity*. He did not move an arm to write a prescription and she did, to give an injection. It is easy to criticise this as a poor way on which to base a moral distinction.

5 Looking at things more fully from the perspective of the doctors' duties reveals few differences. If what is determinative about their duties is to act in the *best interests* of each patient, then Beryl's GP might do so, if only by respecting her autonomous choice about the ending of her life, to pre-empt further suffering. Arnold's GP might have formed the view that his best interests were not served by the prolongation of his life on quality grounds. Both these views are arguable, but accepting that they have force must imply equal moral value in the doctors' decisions.

6 Both doctors have only *accelerated* the natural processes already in progress. Arnold and Beryl would have died fairly soon anyway, and definitive treatment for the primary illnesses (cerebrovascular dementia and metastatic disease respectively) was impossible. Essentially, the doctors did not interfere in the sequence of events brought about by the primary illnesses, but simply altered the time scale.

It might be said that all this is very interesting, and grist to the mill of philosophical argument, but not consonant with everyday practice. A GP might not accede to Beryl's request because it just 'does not feel right'. There is certainly a legal barrier to such an action, but in any event most UK doctors would not agree to the deliberate ending of a patient's life.[3] Doctors who think this way, that it 'doesn't feel right', are representing a school of philosophical thought termed *intuitionism*. It is entirely respectable, though somewhat out of fashion; but it is vulnerable to the charge that 'gut feeling' judgements are inadequately thought-out, or under-theorised.[4] Most GPs, it seems, do acknowledge a moral objection to a lethal injection, although probably less than would object to a non-prescription, and it is necessary to ask why this might be so.

Since the above points can be counter-argued as follows, the acts and omissions distinction does not seem to supply an answer.

1 Foreseeability as described above is irrelevant. What is of relevance is the *intention* of the two GPs. A doctor purposefully and

deliberately sets out to engineer the death of Beryl, albeit with her agreement. The other doctor does no such thing, seeking only to alleviate Arnold's distress or symptoms, and his death is unintended, if at least partially foreseeable. Moreover, a degree of uncertainty attaches to the omission of treatment for Arnold: he might not die, whereas Beryl certainly will.[5]

2   The *outcome* is very different. It cannot be described solely by the death of the patients, being better described by the inclusion of all surrounding events. We could postulate, for example, angry relatives demanding to know why Arnold had not been treated with any treatment possible, whatever his clinical state.

3   *Redefinition* is a descriptive trick. Obviously, if the GP gave attention to Beryl's request, considered it, drew up a syringe of lethal injection, and administered it, she would have been doing so with the full intention of killing her. No weasel words[6] can ignore that reality. The GP omitted potentially life-saving therapy foreseeing, but without intending, Arnold's death. Whilst he may have acted in some beneficent ways, he was inactive in the all-important one.

4   It may not be possible to be held to blame for what we *do not do*. We omit to do many things in our lifetime that we might do, thereby saving lives. We do not, for example, donate our life savings to research into the diseases of the elderly, such that people like Arnold might live longer.[7] Conversely, we can be blamed for actions that are wrong, such as the deliberate ending of Beryl's life. This aspect should be qualified by the observation that where a duty of care does exist, then an omission may be blameworthy: doctors may be failing in their duty by not giving a life-saving treatment to a patient. What defines the failure seems to be the *scope* of the duty. Arguably in Arnold's case the duty did not require life-saving treatment. Arnold's best interests require his doctor to act in a way that minimises his suffering. The omission of life-saving treatment is morally permissible: he will be assured supportive care for as long as he remains alive. Survival at all costs is not necessarily in his best interests. Given a rule against deliberate killing, Beryl's injection is impermissible.

5   *Cause* matters. The GP would have caused Beryl's death by giving a lethal injection, a death which otherwise would have occurred at a later date. The GP did not cause Arnold's death: bronchopneumonia did.

There are several things to notice about these arguments and counter-arguments. Those that are sympathetic to the notion that there are morally significant differences between acts and omissions might say Beryl's GP's actions are not permissible, starting from the premise that deliberate killing is wrong.

In summary, factors assessing the moral value of medical events at life's end are:

- the patient: quality of life
- foreseeability
- intention
- physical movements
- causation
- definition
- outcome.

To be more precise, the distinction between acts and omissions states that taking an intended action leading to the death of a patient is wrong and always must be so. The reliance on the permissibility of some omissions, not necessarily including cases like Arnold's, seems to be secondary to that rule. Someone taking this view would automatically exclude actions such as those of Beryl's doctor, and be more inclined to agree with Arnold's. There is a gradation of permissibility inherent in these cases, which is inconsistent with absolute judgements. Where most doctors find themselves in agreement is with a long-established code of behaviour going back to the time of Hippocrates (*see* Appendix 1):

> I will give no deadly medicine to any one if asked, nor suggest any such counsel

This has since been raised in criminal law to be determinative and is described as follows.

The Doctrine of Double Effect

The ethical principle known as the Doctrine of Double Effect (DDE) looks more closely at the *intention* involved, rather than focusing on the actions or inactions of a doctor, to determine ethical permissibility. It states that a course of action with two possible effects, good and bad, is only permissible if the good effect is the *reason* for so acting and the bad effect is an *unintentional* 'side'-effect. Thus the original action is not intrinsically wrong.

This doctrine has its roots in Roman Catholic teaching and has been widely adopted as a moral justification for actions by people in other cultures as well. Even though the DDE is criticised widely by philosophers on theoretical grounds, the underlying principle governs much of the thinking of doctors and other professionals in clinical practice.

Constance suffered a stroke at 75 years of age, causing a right hemiplegia and dysphasia, with consequent difficulties in her activities of daily living. She lived alone. Seriously ill at first, and at risk of death, she rallied and after discharge from an initial hospital admission, her GP and her community nurse saw her frequently, mobilising full support for her at discharge. Various people called on her at home to aid her rehabilitation, which was slow and incomplete. Speech and language therapists, occupational therapists, care managers, physiotherapists and others all contributed. Constance's demeanour was rather hostile and non-cooperative to all these people but most of them used a cajoling and breezy approach to get her to exercise and improve. Slowly she made progress.

Constance survived her cerebrovascular accident (CVA) by the best efforts of the hospital doctors and began an extended period of rehabilitation. During the course of her hospital stay, no doubt she suffered many uncomfortable tests and investigations. It could be argued under the DDE that the justification for this lies in the 'good' effect of her survival not being outweighed by the 'bad' effect of her residual disability. That was a 'side-effect' of the survival and was proportionate to her gain.

On discharge, the professionals justified their sometimes overbearing encouragement as a 'side-effect' of her overall improvement that was self-evidently a good thing. It was a proportionate balance, they might argue, since use of this technique rather than any other got the best rehabilitative results, despite her occasional distress and avoidance. Furthermore, it was the technique of rehabilitation that caused the improvement rather than her hostility and avoidance.

Dan was a retired railwayman, who had been admitted to a GP community hospital and was in some pain from his terminal liver cancer. The pain had been controlled for some time on simple analgesics and non-steroidal drugs. Latterly, a peritoneal spread of disease brought him unremitting abdominal pain and nausea with vomiting. It was difficult to define his prognosis with precision. His GP commenced treatment with diamorphine and haloperidol via a syringe driver to achieve control of symptoms. He died peacefully 3 days later.

This example is an archetypal illustration of DDE. We will leave aside the observation from palliative care that in fact it is difficult to *prove* that opiates shorten life in terminal illness, and accept for the moment that, in at least some cases, they do.[8]

The moral justification could be argued thus:

- Dan was offered a treatment with two effects: relief of pain (certain) and shortening of life (possible), 'good' and 'bad' effects respectively
- his GP intended only the former, but the latter was a side-effect that was not caused by the action
- given Dan's short life expectancy, the relationship between the two was proportionate
- therefore the GP's actions were morally justified.

This type of reasoning is widely applied in medicine; it is difficult to imagine clinical practice without it, particularly at the end of life. Our observation is that its roots are deep and it underlies the thinking of most doctors as a subtext for decision making.

Compare the case of Beryl with that of Dan. If her GP gives her a lethal injection, she is committing an act that is intrinsically wrong and which is clearly intended. Beryl's death cannot be conceptualised as a side-effect. It is not proportionate to the 'release' she craves that will accompany and define her death. Thus the DDE does not apply and the injection is morally impermissible.

Yet we could argue that an attempt to apply the principle of the DDE to Beryl is dependent on two important factors.

- Beryl's free choice is ignored: any control or responsibility she might have for her own existence is removed. The DDE overwhelms her autonomy.
- DDE depends on accepting 'killing' as an intrinsic wrong in these circumstances. This is a *deontological* moral precept, of Kantian type, where a rule against killing must always be followed.

Criticism of the DDE has focused on the confusion of *foreseeability* and *intention*. As such there is a similarity with the arguments intrinsic to the acts and omissions doctrine already described. Because, for example, the GP could have foreseen that Dan might die sooner as a result of her treatment, that must imply intention, which in turn blurs the distinction between good and bad effects. Thus DDE is undermined and is awkward to operate as a tool of moral justification.

Ordinary and extraordinary treatments

The GP in the first case, that of Arnold, faces a dilemma described in part above. Another way of looking at it is to consider what he might do in terms of possible treatments. At two extremes, he might admit Arnold to hospital (which Arnold cannot resist) where full resuscitative therapy with ventilation, hourly blood gas monitoring, intravenous antibiotics and the full panoply of modern secondary care are set in train, or he might initiate simple supportive treatment in the home. One way of deciding is by according moral value to these possible options. We would say that an 'ordinary' treatment is correct and an 'extraordinary' treatment not so. This distinction requires clarification: 'extraordinary' implies a treatment that is unusually distressing, burdensome or, perhaps, costly.

This was exemplified in a recent case in England, where a 12-year-old girl was refused funding for a second bone marrow transplant for leukaemia, after the first had failed (*see* Chapter 10).[9] From the moral point of view, this second attempt would have been an extraordinary treatment and thus wrong.

Transfer for aggressive treatment in a hospital would be wrong for Arnold on the same grounds. But by this measure, an antibiotic would be classifiable as an ordinary treatment; it is difficult to describe antibiotic treatment otherwise. One of the problems about this ethical rule is definitional. How do we clarify the difference between *ordinary* and *extraordinary?*

There is inevitably an elasticity about describing treatments as burdensome or painful, as one man's burden can be another's benefit and both men can have differing tolerance to these burdens. It is tempting to say that resolution of this aspect depends on the individual patient's own view, as representative of his autonomy. However, if this is accepted, then moral judgements on treatments *per se* are clearly impossible. (*See* Chapter 5 for Pellegrino's comments on illness in general.)

All doctors are familiar with the stoicism of some patients who can bear repeated surgery or chemotherapy in attempts to effect long-term cure from malignancy or even short-term remissions. Others cannot bear such interventions, even when such an outcome is possible. In these situations, the balance between the two scenarios is dependent on the patients, rather than the intrinsic moral value of differing treatments. The notion of ordinary and extraordinary treatments as being morally different is undermined. Moreover, such judgements must often be *context-specific,* which makes a universal approach less easy.

Consider a variation on the Arnold case above.

- Arnold (1) and his GP – as above – conduct their consultation in a well run and supportive residential facility where all possible options can be considered and implemented.
- Arnold (2)'s situation is different. He lives in a run down area with relatives who have looked after him thus far. They are fiercely proud of his survival and pressure the GP very strongly to admit Arnold (2) for aggressive therapy. They brook no argument.

For the relatives of Arnold (2), is it morally right that the life of their family member should be preserved at all costs? Such necessary treatment is not extraordinary. Resource considerations do not enter the frame. For them the *sanctity of life* principle outweighs all other aspects and Arnold (2) is entitled to whatever treatment is necessary to preserve his life, of whatever quality.[10] The doctor might consider such an attitude to be extraordinary but the family do not, and they require his intervention.

In the context of a dispute between family and doctor as to the appropriateness of this intervention, does a moral distinction between ordinary and extraordinary means of treatment help resolve the doctor's problem? It seems not. A more likely means of resolving the dilemma is to consider Arnold (2)'s *best interests*, and whether they are necessarily served by treatment 'at all costs'.

There is another aspect to this area. The assumption so far has been that, if Arnold is not treated 'actively' with antibiotics, he will have supportive care of some type. What might this mean? For example, should Arnold be given fluids orally, or perhaps parenterally, when his illness makes it impossible for him to drink normally? One clinical assumption would be that if this is not done, then he or his relatives might be more distressed than otherwise.[11] The ethical correlate of this position is that hydration is an ordinary treatment, in the terms described above, and thus is morally right for Arnold. More specifically, oral hydration could be considered an ordinary treatment and parenteral hydration not. The elasticity mentioned above seems to return repeatedly when conceptualising moral permissibility on this distinction.

In fact UK law considers any artificial nutrition and hydration as a medical treatment, rather than an ordinary function of basic need or necessity. The *withdrawal* of such treatment in a patient without hope of recovery is lawful,[12] but this is not quite applicable to Arnold, where the problem is deciding whether to *initiate* a line of treatment.[13]

The picture is complicated further by consideration of whether the GP might even add a sedation regime to a decision not to hydrate artificially. If this is done, the moral justification seems to swing closer to the case of Beryl and her GP, though ultimately it would rest on the DDE, or an interpretation of beneficence.

Consider the factors that would make you decide whether to treat Arnold with an antibiotic, or anything else, and why.

The whole picture is neatly summarised by Clough in his oft-quoted phrase:

Thou shalt not kill; but need'st not strive
Officiously to keep alive.[14]

Futility

The nihilist might aver that all human action is ultimately futile, a notion with which few of us would agree, the doctor least of all. It deserves consideration in a discussion of end of life issues because medical decision making often has futility as a subtle background. Implicit in judging a course of action to be futile is a poor likelihood of success, where success is defined as a poor outcome with little health gain.

We could argue that both Arnold (1) and Arnold (2) would undergo futile treatment if admitted to hospital, or indeed treated actively in any sense. If they recovered from their acute illness(es) they would return to a state of profound ill-health from which no further recovery was possible. In doing so, a hospital admission for Arnold (2), under pressure from his family, would involve a great deal of expensive healthcare 'better' applied to someone with a 'better' prospect for more useful recovery, that is to say, doing something more useful such as working, caring for the next generation or creating a great work of art.[15]

Because this view looks to the *outcome* of a possible treatment, it is utilitarian in type. In the case of Arnold, a doctor who invokes the idea of a futile outcome to argue against treatment has acquired the engaging title of a *futilitarian*.[16] It is not possible to avoid bringing a value judgement into any examination of futility. The futilitarian GP treating Arnold (1) would not accept that use of an antibiotic was an 'ordinary' treatment, but would look ahead to what might be left after a successful outcome (in the sense of saving a life). He would speculate that Arnold (1) would remain demented, with little capacity for self-reflection, self-care or self-valuing, and therefore life-saving treatment was futile, though life-prolonging. In reaching this assessment he would accept also that the probability of risk of this outcome was at least more likely than not. Were this not the case, it would not be possible to argue futility. There is, therefore, a descriptive and numerical component to a futility judgement. Perhaps Arnold's GP is such a doctor.

Though the outcome for Arnold (1) might be futile, we must acknowledge that the process of dying (if that is what it is) clearly is not. His doctor facilitates the patient's 'good death' by arranging the other treatments to ease his suffering.[17]

What is euthanasia?

So far this chapter has avoided the use of the term 'euthanasia' but inevitably the word hovers in the background of any discussion of death in medical practice. This avoidance has been purposeful, so as to articulate some of the subjects above in readiness of consideration of euthanasia. Readers will have recognised that Beryl was asking for euthanasia in the commonly accepted use of the word. We need to clarify its meaning.

Euthanasia means a gentle or easy death.[18] Modern usage is consistent with voluntary active euthanasia as outlined below.

Box 9.1   Types of euthanasia 1

Voluntary – patient requests it
Involuntary – patient does not request it
Non-voluntary – patient cannot request it

The first subdivisions of the term encompass the idea of consent to the process. Beryl is *consenting* to her death being brought about by her doctor. It is obviously a voluntary process. By contrast, involuntary euthanasia is tantamount to the judicially defined murder charge, that of premeditated killing with intent. Where consent is not possible then the term non-voluntary is applied, and this refers to situations where people such as newborns or end stage demented patients are allowed to die.

Such subdivisions based on consent overlap those based on process.

Box 9.2   Types of euthanasia 2

Active – either the patient himself, or someone else, takes measures to kill the patient
Passive – no such active measures are taken

Or those based on the interventions of other people, such as doctors or relatives, for example.

Box 9.3 Types of euthanasia 3

Assisted – the patient has help with his death
Unassisted – the patient manages alone

It helps to understand these definitions because it becomes clear that euthanasia involves much greater areas of everyday clinical practice than is at first apparent. All the cases above involve the consideration of euthanasia-related practice.

- Arnold: *Non-voluntary unassisted euthanasia.* By virtue of his inability to consent to treatment options, including non-treatment by potentially life-saving therapy, Arnold was allowed to die, but to do so with caring attention to symptom relief.
- Beryl: *Voluntary assisted euthanasia.* Beryl was in clear consciousness asking for assistance with the process of dying, should the need arise, as she saw it.
- Constance: *Voluntary unassisted euthanasia. In extremis,* a decision might have been made at hospital not to treat her actively, perhaps because a statement to that effect had been found about her person. In this case, we could equally well call this 'rational suicide'.
- Dan: *Voluntary active* euthanasia (if indeed opiates are held to be life-shortening).

Some of these descriptions might appear surprising. This is because it is difficult to apply dry definitions to real cases. Readers may well classify these cases differently and may be right to do so. What is important is the thought about the issues behind the classification as described in the first few sections of this chapter. Some will also have their own views on the moral basis of *voluntary assisted euthanasia,* which is the generally understood meaning of the term.[19]

Legal aspects of euthanasia

As already stated, involuntary assisted euthanasia, because of its non-consensual nature and purposive killing, is unlawful. It is either murder or manslaughter. The concept of 'easy death' is irrelevant.

Further consideration must be given to cases where an easy death is sought by the patient. In only one jurisdiction is this kind of process permitted. Holland allows a defence to the charge of murder where life is actively terminated by a doctor, provided a careful procedure is followed. (Dutch statute law has now been changed.)

There has been much argument as to whether the Dutch are slipping down a slope toward euthanasia of non-voluntary patients and inadequate palliative care on one side or observing a humane attitude to end of life decisions on the other.[20] The fact remains that Holland provides the only framework where cases such as Beryl's are potentially lawful.[21] In England her doctor's action, were the GP to accede to Beryl's request, is unlawful. By contrast, Dan's management is lawful.

That this should be so is best illuminated by the words of the judge in the famous trial of Dr Bodkin Adams in 1957. This GP was charged with the murder of one of his patients who died following the administration of increasing doses of opiates. She had not in fact been terminally ill. During his speech the judge said two things that have entered common law (interpreting statute law) as determinative:

> If the acts done were intended to kill and did in fact kill, it did not matter if a life were cut short by weeks or months, it was just as much murder as if it were cut short by years.

In this phrase, the judge confirms the illegality of Beryl's death. The obvious intention was to comply with her request and end her life. He continued:

> If the first purpose of medicine, the restoration of health, can no longer be achieved, there is still much for the doctor to do, and he is entitled to do all that is proper and necessary to relieve pain and suffering, even if the measure taken may incidentally shorten life.[22]

What is achieved here is the validation of the DDE as a defence in criminal law. The treatment of Dan is lawful as there is no intention to kill, but only to relieve suffering. This assumes that the syringe driver does in fact hasten death. It could be said that the use of a drug like an opiate indicates a therapeutic rather than a lethal intent on the doctor's part.

Things were different in the case of Dr Cox. Readers may already have noted the similarity of Beryl's case to this real one. Dr Cox was a respected rheumatologist dealing with a patient he had known for some time, in severe and refractory pain, and *in extremis*. She requested death repeatedly, and in the end Dr Cox allegedly injected her with potassium chloride, causing death shortly after. As she was cremated, and there was no evidence to confirm the use of potassium chloride, he was charged with attempted murder, and was convicted. In his summing up to the jury, the judge said:

> If he injected her with potassium chloride with the primary purpose of killing her, of hastening her death, he is guilty of the offence charged.

To which a doctor might add that because the injection was potassium and not opiate, the intention is proved. In fact the defence in the trial argued that potassium could be considered an analgesic, without effect.[23]

This is the other side of the DDE: where primary intention is to end life rather than as a side-effect, the action is unlawful, even though moral permissibility is arguable, as above. It might also be observed that the moral principle of DDE risked being circumnavigated by the lack of evidence; in the event, Dr Cox broke the law as evidenced by his conviction as well as the moral principle of the DDE.

Dr Cox was admonished by the GMC and was permitted to practise by his employing authority with certain conditions. This suggests that, despite his conviction, the GMC exercised restraint in his punishment, and were less impressed by the DDE as a moral principle.

This legal framework, despite arguments, is likely to remain with us for some time to come. A recent House of Lords Select Committee on Medical Ethics reinforced the legality of potentially life-shortening analgesia, and the illegality of active euthanasia, so there is little parliamentary impetus for change.[24,25]

Box 9.4   Law and euthanasia

- Intentional killing is unlawful
- The DDE represents the law
- Acts and omissions have legal meaning

Is there a right to die?

As active euthanasia is unlawful it seems that any right to die that we might have is severely curtailed, since those who might assist us are prevented from doing so. Let us examine this more carefully. We will assume that the person wanting to die, like Beryl, is competent and of age. How could her right to die be argued?

Box 9.5   Rights theory: a reminder

- Rights are justified claims on others
- Rights imply obligations on others
- Legal rights are not necessarily moral rights
- Rights may be negative or positive

Beryl has requested the deliberate ending of her life. If her 'right' is to be observed and implemented, this would create a duty to her by her doctor. We might say she has a *moral* right, but clearly she does not have a legal one. Such a right would definitively be *positive* as she wants something done for her. Her qualification as a bearer of such a right rests on her autonomy, which as we have seen elsewhere can in turn be grounded in her understanding, intention and freedom from controlling influences (*see* Chapter 6). Assuming these are present, why should this right not be held to be capable of being realised?

There are two responses to this. First, it could be said that such a right imposes an unacceptable duty on a doctor to make it happen, and currently under law, it cannot. Such a right might also conflict with a doctor's personal moral perspective against deliberate killing.

Second, we might argue that there is no justification for the claim on such a doctor *qua* state. People do not have a basis for engineering their own demise, as life is held to be of value in itself, and the right to die is denied. Put differently it could be said to be against the principle of non-maleficence. However, this is inconsistent with other aspects of law, at least in England.

Suicide is not illegal, but assistance to commit suicide by others is.[26] In contrast, we are permitted to refuse medical treatment for whatever reason, even unto death. So what is brought about is a legal recognition of the difference between acts and omissions, whatever the arguments and counter-arguments at the head of this chapter. It can be described as a modified legal right to *passively* bring about our own demise should we wish it, but not to seek the involvement of others, such as doctors, in actively bringing it about.

Advance statements

These are statements by people requiring or requesting certain forms of treatment or indeed non-treatment, to be applied in future situations when they may not be able to communicate a choice. Such statements are also known as advance directives, or living wills. The legality of advance statements is not in doubt in the UK.[27] Common law on this matter is settled, and following a review of statute,[28] Government is satisfied that the introduction of new legislation is not necessary. Case law in conjunction with the BMA's code of practice provides adequate guidance on advance statements.[29]

Consider a variation on the case of Constance: this note might have been found in her handbag:

To the doctor
    If I ever get really ill and cant speak for myself, like if a have bad stroke or car crash or something and I cant talk and wont get better, please let me die. I don't want to be a burden. God will look after me after I die.

Constance

(sic)

What should community or hospital staff do if they had found such a note when they first saw her? On the face of it, Constance has made a freely autonomous choice predicting her attitude to living with a serious disability, and electing to put her trust in her God instead, requesting the doctors not to initiate treatment but to leave her to die. Perhaps she is exercising a right. But most doctors would hesitate before acceding to her request, and would not implement it.

The principle of beneficence would suggest that she should be treated, against the spirit of her advance statement, on the grounds that there is a reasonable chance of reasonable recovery, and that the chance should be taken. In doing so, staff would be overruling the principle of autonomy, something to be done with considerable caution. Such a course of action is easier for highly trained staff to take whose job it is to make people better, but it is necessary to remember its paternalist basis. A decision to obey the directive would be more difficult to implement. Moreover, there may be a chance of a recovery that would probably be less good if initial resuscitative work was not complete. Such a course of action would not end up being non-maleficent.

In fact, there may be cause to doubt the quality of autonomy at issue here. Constance writes, it seems, with clear intention, but was she aware of the full picture of what rehabilitation can achieve? Was the note written in an atmosphere of coercion created by her relatives? It is not difficult to imagine situations of varying degrees of implied coercion: from direct requests from others in the family to pen such a note, or a general sentiment of non-support of infirm family members. All this would be subsumed under the 'controlling influences' component of autonomy.

Was the note written in full competence? The professionals, who might have known Constance before, might well be impartial observers of this state. The full assessment of competence is dealt with in Chapters 5 and 6 but for the moment we will accept that where there is doubt of this, it is difficult to recognise such a note as being fully autonomous. The text of the note as written betrays no evidence of a psychiatric problem, though it might be argued that the sentiment contained within it is implicit evidence of mental distress.

In summary, what Constance is endeavouring to achieve is a measure of control over her future state, as she predicts it, given certain negative clinical events. To gainsay that control by treating her against those wishes represents a medical decision guided by a paternalistic version of beneficence rather than respect for her autonomy.[30] But it should be noted that from the legal point of view, neither the GP nor the hospital doctors can be required to provide treatment that they do not regard as being in Constance's best interests, whatever her note might say. This is currently under review, and statute to clarify these matters is awaited at the time of writing.[31]

As with consents to treatment, written advance statements are only evidence as to the wishes of the person in question. Morally speaking, a verbal statement carries as much weight, though it would be more difficult to evidence a verbal or non-witnessed written advance statement.

Best interests

One area merits a little more examination in the context of death. The judge in the Bodkin Adams case put it clearly when he referred to the restoration of health as the primary purpose of medicine, a goal with which few would disagree.

But when is that point reached when the restoration of health 'cannot be achieved'? Or put differently, when should doctors palliate rather than cure? The discussion above takes a position as being based upon 'best interests' of the patient. As we have seen this can be interpreted rather differently: Arnold (1)'s GP interprets his best interests as requiring palliation, but Arnold (2)'s relatives see it as life preservation.

Despite this it is obvious that a motive is needed when this vital transition point between active treatment and palliative treatment is negotiated. We have seen that advance statements can guide doctors as to a patient's wishes, as an expression of personal autonomy. The chain of reasoning here is that patients themselves are the best judges of their own best interests in spite of occasional disagreement from doctors.

It should be noted that this principle operates mostly on a negative basis: patients may elect to refuse treatments that can culminate in their death and doctors must follow that choice. But where patients require active treatments that are *not* seen by doctors to be in their best interests, then doctors, at least legally, are not bound to follow patients' free choices.

One reason for this is that an individual's best interests are at least partially dependent on other people's best interests. The case of child B, illuminates this (*see* Chapter 10). If her best interests were defined in her survival, or at least another attempt at chemotherapy directed to this end, other patients in that health authority area would have less resources by virtue of her usage of expensive treatment, thereby compromising *their* best interests. In the event, the court held that her best interests were not served by the burdens of a new chemotherapeutic regime and bone marrow transplant, which had only a small chance of success, and did not approve the treatment.[32]

At the start of life, such decisions are faced in the context of severely damaged newborn infants. Often it is agreed by parents and doctors that a premature infant, born with brain damage and multiple other defects, can be allowed to die and active treatment withdrawn. This agreement represents a coincidence of ethical view between parents and doctors, which amounts to a common acceptance of best interests and quality of life. As we have postulated, this is not always the case, and in recent years the courts have seen a number of cases where they have had to determine the outcome for severely damaged babies.[33]

Generally, it is held that the best interests of these unfortunate infants are not served by their survival, that the potential quality of life renders it more of a burden than not, and that it is lawful to allow death to occur. In doing so, where there is dissent, the courts usually accept the doctors' assessment of 'best interests' rather than the parents'. That fact has not been without adverse academic legal comment.[34]

It is to be regretted that these points of transition were fought over in the courts. It is to be hoped that good communication between doctor, patient and relatives renders all parties as fully informed as possible in order to arrive at an agreed compassionate decision.

Conclusion

This chapter, as well as discussing the ethical aspects of death, has examined some ethical principles other than the four principles and four theories analysis (*see* Chapter 1). What has not been fully examined is the world-wide context. For those who live and work in the West, most of the above discussion will be relevant, and it might be said that Western attitudes to death inform law and ethics in healthcare generally.

Other cultures have different perspectives on death that might inform their healthcare ethics. Stoicism in the face of death is more fully described in Asian societies, for example.[35] However, if the principle of autonomy is regarded as pre-eminent in deciding what is

right in end-of-life issues, and that it is a universally applied principle, then respect for a cultural context is implicit. Nonetheless, as we
have seen, respect for autonomy is not held to be pre-eminent at the
end of life. Ought this to be so?

References and notes

1   Rushdie S (1975) *Grimus*. Panther, London.
2   Illich I (1995) Death undefeated. *BMJ*. **311**: 1652–3.
3   '32% might, according to a survey, and 46% might if it was lawful.'
    Ward B and Tate P (1994) Attitudes among NHS doctors to requests for
    euthanasia. *BMJ*. **308**: 1332–4. Recent general media reports have focused
    on GPs who have ended life deliberately, as described briefly by Dyer C
    (1997) Two doctors confess helping patients to die. *BMJ*. **315**: 206.
4   For a full discussion on intuitionism see Hare RM (1997) *Sorting Out
    Ethics*. Oxford University Press, Oxford, Ch. 5, pp. 82–102.
5   Gillon R and Doyal L (1999) When doctors might kill their patients. *BMJ*.
    318: 1431–3.
6   This phrase is derived from Jaques' 'I can suck melancholy out of a song as
    a weasel sucks eggs'. Shakespeare W *As You Like It*. Act II Scene 5.
7   Such behaviour can be described as 'Good Samaritan' behaviour, mean-
    ing beyond the call of any clear duty. The phrase could be applied to the
    GP here.
8   Expert Working Group of European Assn. for Palliative Care (1996)
    Morphine in cancer pain: modes of administration. *BMJ*. **312**: 823–6 and
    more fully described in Twycross RG (1994) *Pain Relief in Advanced Cancer*.
    Churchill Livingstone, Edinburgh, Ch. 17. This latter book discharges the
    claims that morphine causes individual serious complications such as
    respiratory depression, but not that there is an overall life-shortening
    effect. This would be very difficult to research. It might also be argued
    that life is prolonged by good symptom control.
9   R v Cambridge DHA ex parte B (1995) **2** *All ER*: 129 (the Jaymee Bowen
    case). Part of the reasoning in this case was the experimental nature
    of the treatment which was in itself painful and burdensome to a large
    degree.
10 A useful analysis of the sanctity of life doctrine is in Singer P (1993) *Prac-
    tical Ethics* (2e). CUP, Cambridge, p. 83 *et seq*.
11 This is argued powerfully by Craig G (1999) Palliative care from the per-
    spective of a consultant geriatrician: the dangers of withholding hydra-
    tion. *Ethics and Medicine*. **15**(1): 15–19.

12   Airedale Trust NHS v Bland (1993) *AC*: 789. Tony Bland was a patient in a persistent vegetative state after an injury. As such, he was unaware of his surroundings and state, being essentially decerebrate. Continuation of artificial hydration and nutrition was held not be be in his best interests by their Lordships. Lord Mustill considered him to be without best interests in view of his decerebrate state, but would not have done so had there been 'glimmerings of awareness'.

13   The latest guidance on this subject is from the BMA. British Medical Association (1999) *Withholding or Withdrawing Life Prolonging Medical Treatment: guidance for decision making*. British Medical Journal Books, London.

14   From *The Latest Decalogue* by the poet, Arthur Clough. But as Peter Singer points out, these lines come from a satirical poem that does not advocate any lack of striving. Singer P (1993) *Practical Ethics*. Cambridge University Press, Cambridge, pp. 205–6.

15   This argument explores the value of life. It might be 'instrumental', to mean what life could be used for, or 'intrinsic', to mean of value in itself.

16   Caplan A (1996) Odds and ends: trust and the debate over medical futility. *Ann Intern Med.* **125**: 688–9 and Schneiderman LJ, Jecker NS and Jonsen AR (1996) Medical futility: response to critiques. *Ann Intern Med.* **125**: 669–74.

17   Less dramatic but of equal relevance in the notion of futility is the decision making in favour of palliation that takes place when a malignant disease is past the point of active treatment.

18   *The Concise Oxford English Dictionary* (6e) (1976) reminds us of the Greek roots of this word: *eu-*, well, easily and *thanatos*, death.

19   A full theorisation of the basis of voluntary assisted euthanasia can be found in Keown J (ed.) (1995) *Euthanasia Examined*. CUP, Cambridge.

20   A full discussion is in *J Med Ethics* (Feb 1999) **25**(1). Papers exploring the legal process, empirical evidence of widening criteria for legal euthanasia with a response, and an editorial provide a clear summary of the Dutch experience.

21   Some debate is taking place in Australia. For a six-month period from July 1996, in the Northern Territory, the Rights of the Terminally Ill Act 1995 permitted voluntary assisted euthanasia, and four patients died with assistance, legally. This was revoked by federal legislation later.

22   R v Adams (1957) Criminal Law Reports 365 (CCC) *per* Devlin J.

23   R v Cox (1992) *BMLR*: **12**(38) (Winchester CC) *per* Ognall J.

24   House of Lords (1994) *Report of the Select Committee on Medical Ethics*. HMSO, London.

25   Jeffrey D (1994) Active euthanasia: time for a decision. *Br J Gen Pract.* **44**: 136–8.

26   Suicide Act 1961 ss1 and 2, respectively.

27   Re T (1992) **4** *All ER*: 649.

28 Lord High Chancellor (1999) *Making Decisions.* Lord Chancellor's Department, London, October.
29 British Medical Association (1995) *Advance Statements about Medical Treatment.* BMA, London.
30 A full discussion of this area can be found in McLean SAM (1996) Advance directives: legal and ethical considerations. In: S McLean and I Pace (eds) *Ethics and Law in Intensive Care.* OUP, Oxford.
31 *Who decides?* Chapter 4. This is a UK Government consultation paper on the subject of incapacity and will inform future legislation. The BMA produced *Advance Statements about Medical Treatment* in 1995 as a code of practice for all doctors.
32 The child did have the treatment privately funded but she died in due course.
33 Re C (a minor)(medical treatment) (1998) *Lloyd's Rep Med*: 1.
Re J (a minor: child in care)(medical treatment) (1993) *Fam*: 15.
Re C (a baby) (1996) **2** *FLR*: 43.
34 Medical Law Review (1997) **5**: 102–4 (on the case of Re C (a baby) as above).
35 Maddocks I (1997) Is hospice a western concept? In: D Clark, J Hockley and S Ahmedazi (eds) *New Themes in Palliative Care.* Open University Press, Milton Keynes, p. 195 *et seq.*

CHAPTER TEN

Resource allocation: needs and wants

Summary

This chapter examines the question of rationing in the NHS,[1] and identifies some of the ethical dilemmas and legal issues that it produces.

The complexity of the fair allocation of resources in the health service requires considerable and sometimes inconclusive debate. The important issues to be considered ethically are:

- The patient's view
- The utilitarian view
- The GP as gatekeeper
- Equity and justice
- Rationing and the law.

Let's halve it in three little quarters[2]

Introduction

It has been known for a long time that the NHS budget is finite. No longer can a *complete* 'health service' be available *free to everyone* at the point of contact. Some difficult decisions have to be made on the distribution of available resources, and rationing is inevitable. It is important to include rationing of time, energy and expertise in the discussion; it is not only financial resources that are in short supply, although it is the shortage of funds which is currently foremost in the rationing debate.

There are two main ethical issues that face the GP when considering how best to allocate resources. First, inherent in the individual patient's perceived *need* for treatment is the requirement to respect his *autonomy*, and to *benefit* him with the treatment. Denying him that benefit is unethical. Second, the principle of *justice* takes into account the fact that many other patients and would-be patients have clinical needs. In satisfying the individual, resources are spent and others might not get treatment. Overall benefit to society is reduced, and with a patchwork provision to some individuals and not others, distribution of treatment is inequitable, and therefore unethical.

If we are to recommend a workable ethical system, applicable to everyday general practice, it has to accommodate both elements – the *individual* and the wider *population*. Each patient ought to be treated as an individual. At the same time, each patient will need to understand his own responsibility as a citizen, and not be wasteful with resources such as medicines or the doctor's time.[3]

Rationing

A 'ration' is understood to mean a 'sufficient or adequate amount' of something, a fair portion of the whole. However, the word 'rationing' makes us think of constriction, or scarcity – the restriction of distribution or consumption of a commodity.[4] In healthcare, rationing means that potentially beneficial treatment is provided for some patients yet denied to others. Doctors often find themselves in the position of having to make judgements about treatments, and who gets what. For example, it may not be the availability of an investigation or a treatment that is in question, but its economic cost.

Needs and wants: patient autonomy

We accept that the needs of the individual ought to be balanced with the needs of the general population in an impartial and just way. What do we really mean by 'needs'? For the sake of this discussion, we use the word 'need' to describe 'necessity', and the word 'want' to describe 'desire'. Therefore, 'needs' are clearly identifiable clinical needs, with a requirement for the doctor to respond to symptoms and manifestations of disease; the boundary could be extended to include emotional, psychological, self-limiting or simply patient-perceived needs. Consider the patient who is articulate, vociferous, demanding, or even threatening, when expressing what he considers to be his needs – or necessities. He is likely to have an advantage over the meek and quiescent patient whose clinical needs may be greater. It requires skill and understanding for the GP to remain morally objective in the consulting room.

Does each patient then have the right to express his 'wants' as 'needs', a right that qualifies him to receive all the attention he expects from the system? Or should he be restricted in some way, so that others with an equal right may be treated? Respecting the autonomy of one patient appears sometimes to be in direct conflict with respecting the autonomy of another – which will succeed? The GP faces a fundamental ethical conflict between the individual patient's autonomy and societal justice.

Utility and equity

Ethical dilemmas can arise each time a new effective, but expensive, treatment comes on the market. We have already stated that the NHS budget is finite, and choices will have to be made. Choosing to dispense the new treatment will inevitably mean that some other treatment must be restricted. If restrictions are be placed on availability, either of the new treatment, or of existing treatments, who ought to decide on these? Also, how can the distribution of the treatment be rendered just and equitable? The ethical principle of utility is based on the ideal of maximum benefit for the maximum number. The *utilitarian manager* may consider spreading resources ever more thinly in an attempt to achieve equity for the population.

Professional autonomy and altruism

One of the most difficult ethical dilemmas for the GP is the one that threatens his own professional autonomy and his altruism. Denying care to one patient in order to conserve money for others is difficult to reconcile with his traditional beneficent role. *Moral* objectives, such as the desire to do the best for the patient and the retention of clinical integrity, do not fit easily with rationing of healthcare.

The patient's view

Trust in the doctor[5]

At its best, the relationship between patient and doctor is based on mutual trust (*see* Chapters 2 and 3). The doctor trusts his patient to tell as full and as true a story of his concerns as he can. The patient trusts the doctor to listen, understand and discuss with him choices of treatment, relying on the doctor's medical expertise. In this way, the patient is able to achieve autonomy – his self-determination – and make his decisions accordingly.

There are areas where the doctor's judgement is affected as much by his need to allocate scarce resources as by his wish to treat his individual patient as best he can. If a patient suspects that his doctor is giving him a 'cheap' option without any explanation, his trust in that doctor is likely to be eroded. He may have heard about a new treatment for his condition through friends, the press, or television, and expect the doctor to discuss it as a possibility. How will he feel if, having broached the subject, his GP rejects it out of hand?

Needs and wants: who decides?

A recent example of this dilemma is a useful illustration. An easily administered treatment for a disturbance of normal function came onto the market, heralded by considerable media publicity. The disorder is common but the drug is not cheap. The question arose: is the disorder a medical condition? If so, it could be said that there is a *need* that warrants NHS medical treatment. If, on the other hand, it is not a medical condition, however much a patient *wants* the drug, there is no moral obligation to provide it on the NHS.

Alan and his wife had divorced some years ago. He came to see the GP because, having entered into a relationship with a younger woman, he was experiencing problems with erectile dysfunction (ED). He had planned a surprise weekend trip with his girlfriend and asked the GP to prescribe drug A for him.

Bill had been treated for hypertension for years. He attributed his ED to the drugs he was taking. Although the regimen had been changed several times in attempts to solve his problem, his function was no better. His blood pressure was well controlled, however. He wanted to try drug A.

Colin's mild diabetes had been diagnosed recently, and was now well controlled by oral therapy. Although he had noticed ED for some years before his diabetes was diagnosed, it was the advent of drug A that had given him the impetus to broach the subject of treatment with his GP.

Each of these patients had found the necessary courage to confide their problem to the doctor. The decision to provide or withhold treatment rested with the GP. Two ethical questions arise.

1 Who is morally responsible for accepting or rejecting the individual patient's symptom as a true health need?

Each patient has done his best to describe the problem. Also, he may have gone into considerable detail as to how it is affecting his relationship at home. His distress may have been evident. The GP has the power to relieve that distress. If we view the patient's autonomy as the prime consideration, the doctor has an ethical duty to respond to each individual patient's distress.

It may be that he feels that his duty leads him to prescribe treatment for all such patients. On the other hand, he may consider raising the threshold of 'need', and thus restrict his prescribing.

> 2 If it is a true need, does each patient have an equal claim on resources? If not, is it ethically reasonable for the GP to discriminate between them? And on what grounds does he do so?

Prior to the advent of effective treatment for ED, many men accepted declining function as part of the ageing process – something to be expected. Medical opinion has concurred with this understanding.

But now, with drugs like drug A, the GP has to make an ethical decision whether to continue to agree, or whether to suggest a treatment. Does the advent of a treatment for a hitherto untreatable condition automatically produce a need? If each patient is to be regarded as an autonomous individual, each one will have the right to decide on the use of the global NHS resource. If the patient himself decides to use a fraction of it to attend to what he perceives as a need, we may think that his decision ought to be respected, without further discrimination.[6]

Ethics of media publicity

Most people have access to health information provided by the media – newspaper articles and advertisements, television, and increasingly, the Internet. They do not always realise that those who provide this information may have a vested interest in selling a product, such as drug companies. Although it is illegal to make false claims for an advertised treatment, nevertheless, information is sometimes presented which is biased or incomplete. A patient may become firmly convinced that his condition will be helped by treatment B, and expects his GP to provide it.

> Edna has been overweight for many years. She has tried different weight-reducing diets, lost a few pounds, and each time has put them back on. She is now getting a lot of pain in her knees and back. She has been told that this would happen eventually if she didn't lose weight. She has read the headlines in the newspaper about the new 'fat-buster' drug, and wants to try it.

Edna is convinced that her weight problem is medical, and that it warrants treatment by her GP with this new drug. Her GP, on the other hand, has many patients like Edna on his list. He may fear an influx of similar requests not allowed for in the practice drug budget. He knows that the drug has side effects that may be unacceptable to some patients. He also knows that the drug can be effective in some patients who are prepared to follow the instructions that accompany a prescription, which can also minimise the side effects.

> To what extent is the GP morally justified in trying to play down the media publicity by stressing the drug's unpleasant side effects?

This example is counter-balanced by another where a leaflet was produced as 'an independent view' of treatment for influenza. This gave some facts about the disease, its treatment and prevention, following the arrival onto the NHS drug list of a prescription drug developed to treat the illness. The resource implications of its advent and possible demand for its use were enormous. As the leaflet pointed out in its conclusion: '[t]he benefits, risks and costs of using the medicine across the NHS need to be clarified. For the moment, *Treatment Notes* does not recommend [drug C].' [7]

It is likely that at the time GPs felt that patient information leaflets such as this were helpful in informing the public in a rational way, thus supporting them in decisions to withhold this drug. It would be interesting to conjecture on the individual GP's response to patient information which conflicted with his own ethical values.

The utilitarian view

Aristotle: good achievable by action

Aristotle stated that in all spheres of human activity there will be a good 'achievable by action'. He regarded the 'good' in medicine as *health*.[8] Yet different societies and cultures have different views on the ingredients of health. In the affluent society in Britain, tolerance of physical and mental discomfort is far below that of some other societies, where medical provision is scarce and sporadic, and even in this country there may be variations in expectations of health, and what medicine is able to provide.

Mill: greatest happiness principle

'Utility' was defined by Mill as the Greatest Happiness Principle – promotion of pleasure and freedom from pain. In order to achieve this in the ideal society, each individual had to act in a way that promoted the 'general good'. He referred to Bentham's principle that 'everybody is to count as one, and nobody for more than one.'[9] This *fundamental utilitarian principle* is seen in action in the NHS whenever funds are allocated on a 'per capita' basis. Even if the actual amount is further influenced by loading or minimising factors, it remains a sum calculated according to the population.

Although one individual may express his needs for treatment as paramount, the utilitarian would expect him to 'take his turn' with others in a similar situation. He is only one of many with rights of access to treatment. There is no guarantee that he will take precedence over others where utilitarianism governs. The *classical utilitarian* will not be considering individual expectations, or those of the public, but will be objective and dispassionate when making resource allocation decisions.

Consequentialism

The classical utilitarian will also expect to maximise the 'general good', whilst minimising harm. This is sometimes referred to as the 'consequentialist' approach, in that it is the *consequences* of the decision which must be measured. Thus, when allocating resources, predictions of costs and benefits have to be made and weighed against each other – producing as much good as is possible for the least amount of harm. The public health perspective, and that of the epidemiologist, could be said to use consequentialist principles.

Curing people with effective drugs is good, by contributing to the overall health of the population. Wasting money on futile or ineffective treatment is harmful, as it puts the budget in jeopardy. But in order to use this approach, statements of value must be agreed. The main elements of healthcare that make up the 'general good', and the harms to be addressed, must be declared.

Could the utilitarian principle work in general practice? It has some advantages.

1   Treatment options

Each patient will know exactly which treatments will be available on the NHS, and which will not. He will have access to the reasoning behind each allocation decision. He will be aware that any expectations for treatment beyond that funded would be disappointed. The discussion between him and the GP will focus on *realistic* options of treatment, each being well aware of what is available. There will be no misunderstanding, and the trust between doctor and patient will remain intact.

2   Evidence-based treatment

In order for it to work, it is necessary for the principle to be based on firm evidence of clinical effectiveness for all funded treatments, relying on 'evidence-based medicine'. Thereby the patient will be assured of good quality care. Guidelines on treatment choices will provide information to doctors, who will then be able to apply them to individual patients.

3   Access to treatment

If the principle is applied nationally, geographical ('postcode') variations in access to treatment will be minimised, or even removed, thus satisfying another ethical principle, that of equity. No one person is favoured at the expense of others. More people may be able to have good treatment with benefit to the population as a whole. Indeed, by adhering to the principle of 'the greatest good for the greatest number', utilitarian management of healthcare funds might well satisfy the original aims of the NHS.[10]

Public expectations

There are disadvantages to this system, if it is applied as described. First, provision of healthcare is not quite the same as provision of some other public services. For example, one could expect that emergency services, ambulance and fire, would respond in the same way to similar circumstances, wherever or whoever you are. But if an attempt is made to share out medical treatment to everyone who happens to be in the same circumstances, some needs will be easily satisfied, others not at all. Each patient is an individual with a complex pattern of symptoms. Each will have his own individual level of distress in response to those symptoms. No one person is exactly the same as the next. It could be morally wrong to try to categorise them without including some flexibility to take account of this.

Jane is 44 years old and has been getting hot flushes for a while. She finds her social life is being affected by the symptom. She asks for hormone replacement therapy (HRT) – friends have told her how wonderful it is.

Jenny is also 44 years old, and recently married for the first time. She wishes to start a family but has as yet had no success. She asks for fertility investigations and treatment.

There is clinically effective treatment for each of these women. If successful, the benefit to each individual is clear. But although the overall cost of each treatment is very different, each carries a cost for the NHS. In terms of cost, HRT is relatively cheap, but is Jane expressing a social rather than a medical need? Fertility treatment can be costly but the right to found a family has been identified as a fundamental human right (*see* Chapter 7).

Quality Adjusted Life Years (QALYs)

Health economists have recommended the use of *QALYs* as a method of measuring overall benefit of treatments.[11] As the words suggest, the effect of any particular treatment is measured according to its predicted influence on both length and quality of life. In order to be effective, a treatment must improve the quality of a patient's life at the same time as extending it.

The method invites a compromise between the interests of the individual patient and those of the community, with the former being subordinate to the latter. As Newdick points out, the needs of the individual patient tend to be lost in such a dispassionate calculation.[12] Conversely we could argue that the use of the QALY in resource allocation is truly egalitarian in that it utilises public surveys, thus eliminating the intrusion of different value systems.

Perhaps the inherent ethical problem with the formal QALY principle, if applied to allocation of funds, is its reliance on the measurement of merit, or deserts. It seems too theoretical, cold and devoid of human understanding, intuitively wrong, to apply such measurements to a vulnerable person in order to find out how deserving he is of treatment. But whilst rejecting it as a principle, we have to be honest, and recognise that this is what is already happening, albeit covertly.

In the two examples above, we might anticipate that Jane is likely to get her treatment, but Jenny will have to fulfil some rigorous criteria before she does and is likely to fail on the grounds of age and statistical probability of success.

> In what way will the utilitarian quantify the benefit in treating either or both of these women?

The GP as gatekeeper

Duty to individual patient

The GP is often referred to as the gatekeeper, and as such, the doctor has a moral duty to use resources optimally, with 'diagnostic elegance' and 'therapeutic parsimony'. Here there is no conflict with the patient's good. If financial incentives and disincentives are introduced, they require careful monitoring to be morally acceptable.

They have the potential to lessen the patient's trust in his doctor at the same time as modifying the doctor's freedom to act on the patient's behalf.[13]

> Amy is 14 months old and due for her MMR immunisation. Her mother has read in the press that the jab gives some children autism and bowel disease. She has also read that some GPs are 'throwing off the list' families that refuse immunisations for their children because they lose money for the GPs.

Although the GP may feel able to put a balanced case for immunisation clearly and objectively in the discussion with Amy's mother, her understanding of the GP's argument may be influenced by what she has read.

Duty to practice population and others

Traditionally, the GP has always been the first point of contact for a person who is ill, or who thinks he is ill. At this moment, the person becomes a 'patient'. The GP has a moral duty to that individual to provide medical care as well as a contractual one, under his terms of service. But does the doctor also have a duty to consider other people, and the cost to the system of this person in front of him?

> Frank travels abroad for his firm and has difficulty in adjusting to transatlantic time schedules. He asks for sleeping tablets to use on the plane.

Both Frank and his GP know that he cannot get these tablets without a prescription. The power to provide this is with the GP. He also has the power to decide whether Frank's problem is clinical or social – either way, it is of low priority. He may choose not to issue an NHS prescription, but is prepared to give Frank a hypnotic on the 'black list', whereby Frank will have to pay for his drug.

However trivial it may seem, there is an ethical problem. If we can say that insomnia is a medically treatable condition, and when treated, promotes well-being, how can we then say that Frank's need is only social? Yet many people travel across oceans, continents and time zones without any difficulty. Tablets to prevent malarial infection are not provided by the NHS for travellers, so why should the NHS pay for tablets to ease the discomfort of a long journey? The GP may consider that, in fairness, a principle of *justice* would not provide an NHS prescription for Frank, however small the cost. Yet Frank himself thinks he needs these tablets in order to function properly. If he does not get his NHS prescription, we could say that his *autonomy* is being compromised.

> Which ethical principle will be most useful in guiding Frank's GP?

Value judgements

> Tina's asthma is not responding to simple forms of treatment and a more effective but more expensive treatment is available. But she smokes quite heavily, and has so far resisted all attempts to encourage her to stop: if she did, her asthma would probably be milder.

Tina may already have had a considerable amount of time and effort spent on her problem to no avail. Does her GP 'wash his hands of her', regarding any more resource use as unjustified? After all, he has a responsibility to others who may benefit more from his services and treatment. If he does prescribe more costly medication for her, will it help – and perhaps more importantly, will she comply better with treatment than lifestyle advice? We may consider that Tina herself has a responsibility to look after her own health: if she chooses not to heed her doctor's advice, should we then interfere with her autonomous choice?

It can be difficult to resist the intrusion of value judgements into the process of resource allocation. Should someone who voluntarily destroys their health by the abuse of alcohol, or drugs, or tobacco, or over-eating, have an equal right to treatment of illness provoked by such abuse as another whose lifestyle is temperate? (*See* Chapter 5.) An extreme example is that of liver transplantation for alcoholic liver disease. Donor livers are scarce and liver failure is invariably fatal. It has been argued that those patients needing transplants for liver disease acquired 'through no *fault*[14] of their own' should have a higher priority than the alcoholics.[15]

There are many other less extreme examples which present to the GP. The support and treatment of drug addicts, both for their addiction and for intercurrent illness, can be extremely time-consuming. We recognise that time is a resource: how much time can be allocated to these patients, perhaps at the expense of other patients considered more 'worthwhile'? Also, in making any allocation, is the GP fully aware of the influence his own values have on this? (*See* Chapter 2.)

Prioritising

The range of clinical need among patients will vary from significant to minor. Each one has a 'right' to the doctor's attention, expertise and assistance. It could be said that they do not have equal rights – that there is a hierarchy of priority. But it is also easy to see that this could lead to the introduction of value judgements. It could be that the doctor does not tolerate smokers, especially if they are asthmatic, nor does he empathise with jet-lagged businessmen. Is one person worth spending more time and money on than another? Is self-perpetuated or social discomfort a clinical need that justifies relief from the doctor?

The level of trust within the doctor–patient relationship influences the benefit that any medical intervention might have. There is a dual responsibility – to the individual patient and to society as a whole – and it is important to make this clear to the patient. This is a moral obligation, just as it is a moral obligation to act as advocate for the patient when unacceptable obstructions are placed in the way of beneficial treatment. Yet it would be ethically unacceptable for a GP, as advocate for his individual patient, to manipulate the system to the detriment of other patients.[16] It is important that the doctor's view of what is ethically unacceptable – putting in the balance costs and benefits – is objective and informed.

Professional autonomy

This is variously perceived as paternalism or clinical independence. The doctor, in protecting his professional autonomy, wishes to be in control. Threats can come from outside, from health managers, but also from patients themselves.

> Tina's GP decides to prescribe the more expensive drug for her, and goes to some trouble to explain to her its use and benefits. Yet it becomes clear from her subsequent infrequent requests for repeat prescriptions that she is not using it as prescribed.

The GP may choose to ignore this evidence of non-compliance. Time and trouble has already been spent on her in endeavours to improve her asthma. She has 'wasted' these resources. It could be said that she had disqualified herself from further medical input. Yet her doctor may have mixed feelings to be acknowledged. If he does not pursue the best treatment for Tina, is he punishing her for challenging his control – or is he accepting her right to autonomy, her right to make up her own mind about treatment?

> Which moral argument might justify such a decision by the GP?

Equity and justice

Distributive justice[17]

As a *national* institution, the NHS has to be seen to be fair. The public has a legitimate expectation that healthcare will be distributed equitably, and that inequalities will be minimised and eventually will be removed. In practice, doctors recognise this as an expectation, and, no doubt, their primary care groups (PCGs) will attempt to satisfy it within the confines of their budget allocation. They will be helped by the growing public understanding that the NHS cannot pay for everything for everybody all of the time. Nevertheless, resource allocation decisions have to be made by somebody, based on the principle of distributive justice.

Fair shares

The political philosopher John Rawls, when discussing *distributive justice*, describes his concept of the 'veil of ignorance'. The rational and self-interested members of a society agree principles of justice, without contamination by personal or public agendas, a state of 'mutually disinterested rationality', of impartiality.[18] The resulting social contract would protect the weakest members of society from further disadvantage: when drawing up such a contract, how can we be sure that we will not have need of support in the future? So we include provision for that support in our plan. Each individual chooses how shares are to be distributed and society will be responsible for guaranteeing the individual fair shares.

Individual freedom

An alternative view is put forward by Robert Nozick. He is concerned that a pure egalitarian principle, such as that described by Rawls, produces a very restrictive society where individual freedom is compulsorily limited. This would entail continual interference, both with those distributing resources, and with those receiving them, in order to maintain a balance.[19] He is a fierce defender of the rights of the individual, and of the protection of these rights against the activities of the state. His concept of equality depends on the right of each individual to 'spend' the resources attached to him according to his own wishes.

The concept of distributive justice is very deeply rooted in us. Some differences between individuals or groups of individuals are morally irrelevant. Beyond these differences, there are others, which might lead to differences in the distribution of 'goods', and this is where disagreements occur. Equality, needs, effort, talents, each is based on the concept of justice. But what about the market? Here there are a number of different values that are obtained when considering distribution, liberty and utility. Rawls' view of liberty and utility, by including this in a concept of justice, is a muddled way of looking at it. It is an attempt to reconcile these two very different sets of values, an attempt which does not work. One can recommend the pluralist view instead, using analysis, reasoning, and balancing conflicting argument.

Who is to make these decisions? Nozick's idea of the 'individual with rights' would be difficult to accommodate in a state-funded system such as the NHS. Should the public have the power through the democratic process? But democracy is by no means perfect. And what about sections of society who cannot vote, for whatever reason? The tyranny of the majority does not protect the minority.

Aristotle had his own view of distributive justice. Inequality is the source of disagreements, and awards, or 'shares', must be allocated according to merit. He stated that this was generally agreed among men, although the elements of merit would still need to be specified:

> This is the origin of quarrels and complaints – when either equals have and are awarded unequal shares, or unequals equal shares ... awards should be 'according to merit'; for all men agree that what is just in distribution must be according to merit in some sense ...[20]

> A GP practice has allocated £x per year for a certain treatment. Which is more ethically sound:
>
> (a) to spend the money on a first come first served basis or
> (b) to institute a points system to choose who gets the treatment and who does not?

Each choice has its disadvantages. If (a) is chosen, how are those patients to be treated who arrive with their problem after all the money has been spent? It would have been impossible to predict whether they had a greater clinical need than those already treated, but suppose this was the case? Do they wait in a queue for the beginning of the next financial year? If on the other hand (b) is chosen, how are points to be allocated, and on what degree of clinical need is the decision to be based? The money may still run out before the year end – or there may be some left over. There may, of course, be a third choice, (c), where pragmatic decisions are made on a case-by-case basis. This will rely heavily on the doctor's 'mood of the moment', and apart from allowing gross paternalism, could not be said to be fair.

Mill introduced the idea of expediency. Social inequalities which are not expedient, or which become inappropriate in their context, are injustices.[21] If this maxim is to be used in the NHS context, we need to define a 'recognised' expediency, and to decide whether a cash shortage can be an ethical justification for inequalities of treatment. We could plead 'expediency' where a treatment is refused because the budget is overspent. Any moral concern ought to be directed towards the fundamental reasons for overspending: was the budget too limited, and was its level unchallenged? Had the money been misspent, or wasted?

Michael has had low back pain for a few days, since laying some paving stones at his home. The pain has not stopped him doing anything and he has not stayed home from work. He wants to be pain-free for a golf match next weekend and has already tried drug C from a friend, which is 'marvellous'. He asks his GP for a prescription. Drug C is the most expensive in a range of drugs used for back pain, and has not been shown to have any advantage over the others in clinical trials. However, he maintains that he has tried the others in the past and they were 'useless'.

Michael is a tax-payer and, using Nozick's recommendation, ought to be able to 'spend' his personal NHS budget as he chooses: after all, he has paid into the system for many years through his taxes. He expects to realise his right to medical care. His GP has a contractual duty towards him to provide such care. The GP also knows that a patient's past experience (Michael's reference to the uselessness of other drugs) may influence his clinical response to a proposed alternative. But the GP has a duty not to be wasteful. Using drug C would be wasteful, if another drug would perform the function just as efficiently.

Does the GP assume total responsibility for saying 'no' to drug C, prescribing the cheaper alternative? Does he go further by giving Michael factual information on comparative efficacy and costs of the drugs? Or does he decide that Michael's attendance for a minor self-limiting condition is not appropriate and recommend an over-the-counter remedy?

Rationing and the law

Whatever the ethical position might be, patients have little recourse in law when they experience difficulty in obtaining medical treatment because of its cost to the NHS. If this is unreasonable, what are the realistic alternatives? If a GP's treatment for his patient conflicts with restrictions imposed by a funding authority, can this be regulated, referring to the GP contract and his duty of care? Allocation of drug budgets has now been devolved to PCGs. At the same time, so-called 'postcode' variations in access to treatment have become overt.

The GMC's requirements for good practice do not necessarily match with resource limitations and rationing, particularly with the influx of new and effective prescription drugs. The public has been assured of the protection of the GMC in quality and performance issues; it is unclear whether this can go further and address the conflicts produced by rationing of resources.

Healthcare law, and in particular, the provision of medical services, is based on rules governing the practice of health professionals.[22] GPs practise according to their terms and conditions of service.[23] They are also bound by the GMC, which, if it finds a GP guilty of malpractice, can suspend or remove him from the medical list, thus forcing him out of practice. It could be said that if a patient *needs* treatment with a drug licensed for his medical condition, refusing to prescribe the drug could not be 'good practice'.

The GP Contract

Many symptoms are unpleasant and can occur with no diagnostic evidence of disease. Patients bring to their GPs common everyday problems, and also an expectation that the GP will provide them with relief. Satisfaction or rejection of the expectation of a prescription or treatment provision rests with the doctor using his clinical judgement.

A GP has a direct duty of care to those on his NHS list. This duty, to treat 'appropriately' and to provide prescriptions 'needed' by the patient, is an unequivocal statement governed by statute under the Terms and Conditions of Service.[23] It is the 'duty to prescribe' and the interpretation of clinical 'need' where a problem may lie, particularly if the patient and doctor are not in agreement. As we have seen, the distinction between a need and a want can be interpreted in different ways by different people. In law, the question of needs or wants could be resolved on the basis of either *Bolam*[24] or *Wednesbury*,[25] depending on whether it was a clinical- or a resource-based problem.[26]

The GP must provide 'personal medical services'[27] to his registered patients, although such services are not *absolutely* defined in the regulations. The Patient's Charter expands on them, stating ten rights of the NHS patient. It refers to the right to be registered with a GP for primary care, and to receive healthcare on the basis of clinical need rather than the ability to pay.[28] It does not place the dissatisfied patient in a better position if he wishes to challenge a refusal of treatment in the courts. In law, the two routes open to him remain: using public law by way of judicial review, or civil law claiming negligence. His only other recourse is through the NHS complaints procedure, direct to the GP's practice.[29] If this fails to satisfy him, he can appeal to the Health Service Commissioner (HSC).

The General Medical Council (GMC)

The GMC is the body regulating the registration and professional conduct of doctors (*see* also Chapter 2). It has specific powers under the Medical Act 1983: which 'shall include the power to provide, in such manner as the Council think fit, advice for members of the medical profession on standards of professional conduct or on medical ethics.' If the GMC finds a doctor guilty of professional misconduct, it will impose one of a range of sanctions. The most severe of these is the removal of that doctor's name from the Medical Register so that he can no longer practise.[30]

It states clearly that 'good clinical care must include an adequate assessment of the patient's condition, providing or arranging treatment as necessary' with the proviso that '[i]n providing that care doctors must pay due regard to efficacy and use of resources, and prescribe treatment that serves the patient's needs'.[31]

Information for patients

A doctor's duty of care includes the provision of enough information to enable his patient to make an informed decision on which treatment option to choose. If the doctor anticipates that it is unlikely that his patient will accept the cheapest option merely on the grounds of cost-benefit, he may be less inclined to include that part of the argument.

> [P]atients when insistent are probably more likely to receive the interventions they seek because typically doctors are uncomfortable with the tensions these patients introduce. This is particularly so when the intervention at issue is seen as efficacious but there is just not enough to go round.[32]

The BMA has sought to emphasise this point.[33] Having said that doctors feel reticent, or even 'acutely embarrassed' when discussing funding problems with patients, it advises that:

> [t]he public should be helped to gain awareness, in general terms, of issues of funding and rationing in the NHS. Concern has sometimes been expressed that clinical evidence about the efficacy of some procedures is not being widely disseminated due to lack of funding.

If a treatment is being withheld on grounds of cost, it is clear that the law on informed consent requires the doctor to tell the patient that this is so. A patient refused treatment by his doctor on what he understands to be clinical grounds will naturally feel aggrieved if he later discovers that this was only part of the truth. Of course, if cost was the only reason for the refusal, and the patient was not privy to this, the doctor could then be said to have acted with 'bad faith'.

> Peter, a newly registered patient, asks for a repeat prescription for his dyspepsia. He tells the new GP that he found drug A effective for his symptoms, but his previous GP had changed him to drug B. He says he was told that the reason for the change was that drug A could cause cancer and drug B was safer. He agreed to the change. But drug A and drug B have the same side effect profile, each with the same minuscule risk of cancer. Drug B is cheaper than drug A.

Was this a case of withholding information in bad faith? The ethical viewpoint of the previous GP seems to be in question, yet the law might say that the patient had not suffered harm nor was there a trespass, thus absolving the GP from blame. In *Chatterton* Judge Bristow said: 'in my judgement it would be very much against the interests of justice if actions which were based on a failure by the doctor to perform his duty adequately to inform were pleaded in trespass'.[34] In this case, the first GP had informed Peter of the small risk of cancer with drug A but the patient was not aware of the similarity between drug A and drug B. However, this information would have been available to him in a leaflet enclosed with the dispensed product. Such a leaflet is very comprehensive and its provision is governed by statute.[35]

The GMC regards the provision of information to patients as an important aspect of the maintenance of trust between doctor and patient (*see* Chapter 2). 'To establish and maintain that trust you must ... give patients the information they ask for or need about their condition, its treatment and prognosis.'[36] Although there may be a professional and moral judgement to be made in this case, there would be no realistic legal sanction.

Resource allocation and case law

The Government knew that the NHS would be inheriting resource problems when it was set up in 1948. Hospital facilities were inadequate and unevenly distributed, there were shortages of nurses and doctors, and GPs had to be compensated for the loss of value of their practices. Clement Attlee observed: 'We shall have to be a bit lenient with the service at first.'[37]

Perhaps unintentionally, this 'leniency' was observed for some years, and litigious tendencies were restrained. It was over 30 years before protests from patients about allocation of resources reached the courts. There has been a steady flow since then. An analysis to show the way the law may develop has been suggested,[38] which is of interest when we place it beside the ethical discussion.

1 The benchmark situation.

This measures the level of care provided against a reasonable standard. If the care does not reach this level, there is a breach of duty. The problem with this is where the defence relies on the plea of lack of available resources, and the court has to decide whether to accept this argument. In *Wilsher*[39] a premature baby was in the care of junior doctors, following which the baby suffered damage to his sight. In the Court of Appeal, the wider question of resource allocation was posed by Judge Browne-Wilkinson.

> Given limited resources, what balance is to be struck in the allocation of such resources between compensating those whose treatment is not wholly successful and the provision of required treatment for the world at large? These are questions for Parliament, not the courts.[39]

Although the judges recognised that lack of resources may have been a factor in this case, they were reluctant to base any judgement, even in part, on that aspect. This was not considered to be the court's responsibility.

2 Non-provision of care

Here the court decides whether absolute failure to provide a service is justified, relying on what is reasonable in the circumstances as presented. It could find difficulty in challenging a policy decision by an authority. In 1980, four people sought a declaration that the Secretary of State had failed in his duty to provide a comprehensive health service. They had all been waiting for orthopaedic surgery for some years from their local hospital, and felt they had been waiting long enough. It was put to the judges that the Secretary of State had a duty under Section 3(1) of the National Health Service Act 1977 'to provide ... to such extent as he considers necessary to meet all reasonable requirements ... (f) such other services as are required for the diagnosis and treatment of illness.' But Lord Denning rejected the argument put by the plaintiffs that '[i]f the Secretary of State needs money to do it, then he must see that Parliament gives it to him. Alternatively if Parliament does not give it to him, then a provision should be put in the statute to excuse him from his duty.' It is interesting to note the ground on which he based his rejection.

> It cannot be that the Secretary of State has a duty to provide everything that is asked for in the changed circumstances which have come about. That includes the numerous pills that people take nowadays: it cannot be said that he has to provide all these free for everybody.[40]

The Secretary of State has an obligation to promote a comprehensive free health service under the terms of the National Health Service Act 1977[41] in spite of Lord Denning's colourful interpretation of this duty. However, an application for judicial review of a health authority's decision to refuse assisted fertility to a woman on the grounds of her age failed, although she had based her application on the duty of the Secretary of State.[42] Grubb comments:

> Given that the authority's policy was overtly based upon its need to allocate limited resources, the outcome was almost inevitable. The courts have eschewed involvement in cases concerned with

the allocation of resources within the health service . . . It was not a case where court was concerned to consider denial of access to IVF treatment other than on the basis of financial constraints.[43]

In another case the health authority refused to fund the drug beta interferon for a multiple sclerosis patient. Funds were available but the health authority chose not to spend them on this case. Its specious argument was rejected by the judge as *Wednesbury* unreasonable.[25] The court stayed clear of considering the resource allocation question, as this was seen to be non-justiciable. However, as Newdick points out:

> [t]he case demonstrates that the intractable problems of allocating scarce health service resources are not the unique responsibility of health service managers. The reasons given for their decisions must be candid, consistent, and cogent. It would be wrong, however, to think that the case provides patients with greater access to expensive medicines.[26]

In contrast, a recent case in the High Court demonstrates a change of attitude in the courts. Judge Hidden ruled that a health authority's decision not to fund sex change surgery for three transsexuals was 'unlawful and irrational'.[44] He rejected the health authority's plea that it was entitled to take into account the issue of scarce resources when deciding not to fund these operations. He pointed out that such a restrictive policy would affect any duty to provide treatment for 'the prevention of illness and care of persons suffering from illness'. Vivienne Nathanson, head of science and ethics at the BMA, is quoted as saying:

> it could mean that there are significant limits on what the NHS can refuse to make available. It could mean that if something is a recognised medical condition with a recognised medical treatment, the NHS has to offer that. The implication is that the NHS could not say that new and expensive treatments would not be available.[45]

The judge in this case was clearly persuaded that surgery for gender reassignment was 'proper treatment for a recognised illness'. His judgement reflects an opinion that the plaintiffs were suffering from an illness. It has been upheld in the Court of Appeal, where the judges found that the health authority had exerted a 'blanket policy' while claiming to consider each case on its merits.

Although the appeal court accepted that health authorities are forced to ration treatment where resources are limited, nevertheless, the grounds on which such rationing decisions are made must be based on lawful and proper assessment of the conditions competing for treatment. This is an important decision which is likely to inform court decisions on inequity in rationing in the future.

3   Curtailed provision

These cases have arisen as a result of 'cut-backs' in services previously provided by health authorities. Although in theory they may be considered as starting from a different point than those based on non-provision of services, the problems they pose are similar. The plaintiff complains that medical treatment has not been provided for a medical condition, due to failure to allocate resources. If the health authority had undertaken to provide a certain standard of service and was now providing the same service to a lower standard, for example to fewer patients in their population, or with longer waiting times for treatment, in order to save money, this would be a curtailment.

A particular case attracted a considerable amount of publicity in the media. 'Child B' had already been treated for leukaemia, and the disease had recurred. Further treatment was refused, ostensibly on clinical grounds, but there were also financial considerations. There was an attempt by Judge Laws in the High Court to make the health authority justify its decision, which would have been a step forward in making resource allocation decisions more transparent, being a 'legitimate public law approach, concerned with the process of decision making'. Sir Thomas Bingham, on appeal, rejected this approach. 'Difficult and agonising judgements have to be made as to how a limited budget is best allocated to the maximum advantage of the maximum number of patients. This is not a judgement that the court can make.' The Court of Appeal preferred to judge the issue on what was given as the main reason for refusing treatment, that of clinical opinion. It did not consider that the resource allocation issue was a significant part of the argument, and may have regarded it as non-justiciable.[46]

New treatments are now being introduced at frequent intervals. For example, in vitro fertilisation (IVF), at first controversial, is now accepted as a treatment for infertility. The legal system has been closely involved. As the Canadian Law Reform Commission's recommends: '[l]egislation governing access to medically assisted procreation technologies should respect the right to equality. Access should be limited only in terms of the cost and scarcity of resources.'[47]

This reference deals with infertility treatment, but it describes reasons for rationing which apply to any effective treatment to which access may be limited for resource reasons. No one denies that the NHS is unable to bear the cost of every available treatment for everyone that wants it. Difficult decisions on allocation have to be made. It is important that these decisions are fair, and that patients have their access to treatment upheld by the legal system.

Conclusion

Although the problem of rationing is a complex one, it cannot be ignored in the hope that someone else will sort it out. Every patient consultation with a GP has a resource cost; and each decision on the use of resources has an ethical dimension. Clarifying what *ought* to be done will enable the GP to understand how well (or badly) he is doing in his efforts to reach the moral objective. Equity will best be served by using good information to choose cost-effective treatments that will contribute most to the aim of the NHS – maximising health. Within this framework it is important to take account of people as individuals, each one of value as a person and each one with an *equal* claim to healthcare.[48]

References and notes

1   Peter Singer refers to rationing as 'priority setting' and describes a framework for *accountability for reasonableness* developed by Daniels and Sabin. Singer P (2000) Medical ethics. *BMJ.* **321**: 283.
2   Overheard in children's playground.
3   Broken appointments with GPs are said to cost the NHS £200 000 per year according to a survey by Professor Francome of the Department of Medical Sociology at Middlesex University.

4 Hall MA (1994) The ethics of health care rationing. *Public Affairs Quarterly.* **8**(1): 33.
5 There are parts of this book where issues need to be repeated. The reader will find that **trust** is an important example.
6 The Government restricted the prescription of Viagra on the NHS to men with certain specified medical conditions in a series of circulars, the last in June 1999. The General Practitioners Committee (GPC) of the British Medical Association (BMA) expressed concern that 'most patients with clinical needs equal to those who will receive NHS Viagra will either be denied treatment or have to purchase it privately.' GPC (1999) *Viagra – The Rationing Debate.* BMA House, 29 January.
7 *Treatment Notes* (January 2000) Consumers' Association, London.
8 Aristotle (1925) *The Nicomachean Ethics.* Oxford University Press, Oxford.
9 Mill JS (1962) *Utilitarianism.* HarperCollins, London, p. 319.
10 *National Health Service Bill* second reading, House of Commons, 30 April 1946.
11 Williams A (1985) The economics of coronary artery by-pass grafting. *BMJ.* **291**: 326–9.
12 Newdick C (1995) *Who Should We Treat.* Oxford University Press, Oxford, pp. 26–9.
13 Pellegrino E (1998) Rationing health care, the ethics of medical gatekeeping. In: JF Monagle and DC Thomasma (eds) *Health Care Ethics.* Aspen, USA.
14 Author's italics.
15 Moss AH and Siegler M (1991) Should alcoholics compete equally for liver transplantation? *JAMA.* **265**(10): 1295–8.
16 Tavistock Group (1999) A shared statement of ethical principles for those who shape and give health care. *BMJ.* **318**: 249–51.
17 It is important to distinguish this from *retributive justice* meted out to convicted criminals by the law on behalf of society.
18 Rawls J (1972) *A Theory of Justice.* Oxford University Press, Oxford.
19 Nozick R (1974) *Anarchy, State and Utopia.* Blackwell, Oxford.
20 Aristotle (1925) *The Nicomachean Ethics.* Oxford University Press, Oxford.
21 Mill JS (1962) *Utilitarianism.* HarperCollins, London.
22 Montgomery J (1997) *Health Care Law.* Oxford University Press, Oxford.
23 National Health Service (General Medical Services) Regulations 1992, No. 635 Sch. 2 paras 12 & 43.
24 The Bolam test is derived from a case in 1957, Bolam v Friern HMC. 'A doctor is not guilty of negligence if he has acted in accordance with a practice accepted as proper by a responsible body of medical men skilled in that particular art.'
25 In legal terms, decisions are *Wednesbury* unreasonable if they are so unreasonable that no reasonable person addressing himself to the issue

in question could have come to such a decision. *See* also Newdick C (1996) *Who Should We Treat.* Oxford University Press, Oxford, p. 125.

26 Newdick C (1998) The health care system. In: I Kennedy and A Grubb (eds) *Principles of Medical Law.* Oxford University Press, Oxford, p. 52.

27 A phrase not to be confused with the 'PMS' scheme currently being piloted.

28 Department of Health (1995) *The Patient's Charter.* HMSO, London.

29 National Health Service (General Medical Services) Amendment Regulations 1996, SI No. 702, s47A.

30 Medical Act 1983 part V ss 35 & 36.

31 General Medical Council (1998) *Good Medical Practice.* GMC, London, p. 3.

32 Mechanic D (1995) Dilemmas in rationing health care services: the case for implicit rationing. *BMJ.* **310**: 1655–9.

33 British Medical Association (1997) *Duty of Candour? Truth Telling and Rationing of Resources.* BMA, London.

34 Chatterton v Gerson (1981) *All ER* 257.

35 Medicines (Leaflets) Regulations 1977, SI 1977 No. 1055.

36 General Medical Council (1998) *Good Medical Practice.* GMC, London, p. 5.

37 On this day: Attlee outlines plans for NHS *The Times* **5 July 1999**.

38 Kennedy I and Grubb A (1994) *Medical Law: text with materials* (2e). Butterworths, London, p. 420.

39 Wilsher v Essex AHA (1986) **3** *All ER*: 801.

40 R v Secretary of State for Social Services ex p Hincks (1980) **1** *BMLR*: 93 (CA).

41 National Health Service Act 1977 part I s1.

42 R v Sheffield Health Authority ex p Seale (1994) **25** *BMLR*: 1 (QBD).

43 Grubb A (1996) Infertility treatment: access and judicial review. *Medical Law Review,* p. 327.

44 R v North West Lancashire Health Authority ex parte A and others (1998) *QBD.*

45 Dyer C (1999) Transsexuals win case for NHS funded surgery. *BMJ.* **318**: 75.

46 R v Cambridge District Health Authority ex p B (a minor) (1995) **1** *FLR*: 1055 (QBD).

47 Kennedy I and Grubb A (1994) *Medical Law: text with materials* (2e). Butterworths, London, p. 784.

48 Culyer AJ and Harris J (1997) Maximising the health of the whole community. *BMJ.* **314**: 667–72.

CHAPTER ELEVEN

Looking forward: the advance of ethics in general practice

There is no timeless, unalterable concept of justice or property or freedom or rights – these values alter as the social structure of which they are a part alters . . .[1]

In the past, doctors have relied upon the framework provided by Hippocrates. The Hippocratic Oath concentrates on the doctor and his behaviour towards others. His view of the patient is protective and paternalistic: there is no recognition of a patient's autonomy. The importance of respect for autonomy, or self-determination, is an ethical viewpoint that has developed only recently and on which much ethical argument now rests. This example demonstrates how subsequent developments in moral theory have influenced medical ethics through the centuries: Aristotle, Kant, Mill and the modern philosophers have all contributed in their writings with ideas on virtue, duty, utility and rights. There are many possible developments in medical practice that are likely to require ethical debate. What might the future hold, and will these philosophical tenets continue to provide a useful basis for ethical decisions?

If we look into the 'crystal ball' we can see that some of these developments will be particularly relevant to the GP:

- the Human Rights Act
- litigation
- public expectations and demand
- allocation of resources

- the individual citizen's responsibility
- evidence-based practice
- genetic screening
- euthanasia
- the new NHS
- the future GP.

The Human Rights Act

The passage and implementation of the European Convention of Human Rights is likely to provide a new legal framework for the UK. The language of rights has not so far permeated UK law to any degree, in contrast to some other jurisdictions. In the USA, for example, the original Supreme Court decision that in effect legalised abortion was founded on the pre-eminence of privacy rights. In the UK a similar position was arrived at by the passage of an Act of Parliament which used risk of harm to establish legal justification. Future court decisions in the healthcare arena will have to take into account the new Act.[2]

What effect could this have on ethical decision making? On the one hand many complex ethical decisions might be legally reinforced by the Human Rights Act with benefit to individuals. On the other hand there is a possibility that in adhering to the legal precepts in the Act ethical choices might be restricted in some way for some people, enhancing without resolving the familiar tension between the rights of the individual and those of the wider community.

The sections of the Human Rights Act 1998 that have relevance to healthcare are listed in Appendix 4.

Litigation

GPs are less likely than hospital doctors to have a claim made against them upheld in the courts.[3] Yet many GPs would admit to a fear of this happening, however assiduously they commit themselves to 'good medical practice'. This is in spite of the genuine reluctance of patients to complain about their own GP, someone whom they have known and trusted and whose judgement they have respected over many years.

A change in the manner in which primary healthcare is delivered may have an important effect on the volume of complaints. It is foreseeable that a fragmentation of responsibility in primary care will dilute the sense of continuing personal care currently provided by the GP. Where individual patient care is provided concurrently by several different health professionals, as is happening more and more, cohesive care will rely upon good communication between the professionals themselves and with the patient. There is more opportunity for problems to arise, a dissatisfied or damaged patient to result, and subsequent litigation.

GPs will have to decide how to achieve clinical and ethical continuity in the face of the fear of increasing litigation. The natural response is to practice 'defensive' medicine; this is not necessarily ethically sound, being wasteful of resources and possibly maleficent towards the patient, subjecting him to clinically unnecessary and intrusive investigations.

Public expectations and demand

There are increasing demands on healthcare provision being made by the public in terms of freedom of access, use of new technology and drugs, as well as detailed information on risks and benefits of treatment. The ultimate expectation appears to be the achievement of perfection. It is an onerous task to fulfil such demands and expectations, particularly within the confines of a state-administered healthcare system. The ethical principles governing autonomy and justice will often be in conflict, a conflict that will need to be resolved by GPs as well as all other doctors.

Allocation of resources

The recent changes in the administration of primary care have widened the role of GPs in deciding access to new drugs as well as to secondary care. Priorities will have to be set in a way that is ethically sound. This process will need a recognisable framework for legitimate and fair decisions and as Peter Singer proposes, an 'accountability for reasonableness'. He describes the framework put forward by Daniels and Sabin:

- publicity – decisions and rationales to be publicly accessible
- relevance – to the needs of the population to be covered
- appeals – a mechanism for challenge and resolution of dispute
- enforcement – volutary or public regulation.

As public expectations increase and new technology and treatments are developed, so the need for such reasonableness will assume more importance.[4]

The individual citizen's responsibility

How much will personal responsibility determine access to health-care? Each citizen has a right to healthcare, but with each right there comes a responsibility. This responsibility includes the proper use of resources by the patient: medicines, the GP's time and exper-tise. It could be argued that there is also a more fundamental respon-sibility for each individual to care for and to preserve his or her own health and to resist any indulgence in activities proven to be detri-mental to health. Smoking, alcohol and drug abuse are examples of such activities. Should dangerous sports be included in this?[5]

There is little evidence at the present time that these important aspects of individual and public responsibility are being addressed. Does the GP have an ethical duty to improve public awareness of individual responsibilities to reduce wastage of healthcare resources and damage to health?

Evidence-based practice

Good medical practice is becoming more reliant on a sound evidence base. In ethical terms this could be considered as a virtuous process by which the general (population-based studies) is brought to the particular (the individual patient). Where evidence-based medicine scores highly is in enhancing the GP's ability to explain the clear validated evidence base for the success or otherwise of a particular treatment and to present to the patient the known risks and benefits. Doctors who make idiosyncratic decisions are marginalised by this system, since such decisions have not been subject to rigorous testing. Yet there are many who consider that evidence-based practice and strict adherence to protocols impose unacceptable restrictions on the choices available to individual patients. How will the profession and the law deal with doctors who behave idiosyncratically? On the other hand, the behaviour of many GPs is inherently untestable; can the effect of compassion and courtesy be tested quantitatively?

Genetic screening

It is now possible to identify the genes responsible for the development of some diseases. The advance in this technique is likely to continue. Genetic screening for an increasing number of abnormalities has the potential for affecting actuarial predictions of continuing health and life expectancy. Already this is influencing the actions of insurance companies. The effect may be more widespread in the future when considering procreative choices. Is there an ethical duty to protect future generations from harm by directing fertility away from the 'imperfect'? The utilitarian would argue that the promotion of good and the prevention of pain would be well served by the avoidance of procreation of possible 'miserable' imperfect individuals.

Yet any moral justification for this proposal removes the right of existing 'imperfect' individuals to respect as human beings of value. The intuitive fear of a policy of eugenics arises almost immediately. It would be morally repugnant to destroy such individuals after birth. At what stage, before birth or before conception, does it cease to be repugnant to engineer the constitution of future populations? [6]

Euthanasia

The debate continues towards the clarification of the 'right to die'. There is no legal possibility of euthanasia at the present time. Is the continuing application of the doctrine of double effect ethically useful to the dying and their GPs? It appears to remove the legal threat from the doctor, but increasingly there are concerns voiced by individual patients who dread an inevitable disastrous helpless situation, such as those suffering from motor neurone disease. They wish to demonstrate their self-determination by giving the doctor the responsibility of ending their lives at that point in the future. Will such an action on the part of the doctor be carried out with compassion, or will doctors continue to feel a natural resistance to such intentional killing?

The new NHS

There are considerable tensions between public expectations of a national health service and government provision of resources for such a service; these are likely to continue as long as the NHS remains politically controlled. Any attempt by government to resolve these tensions is likely to have an effect on the way that GPs work.

Traditionally, the GP has considered the individual patient's needs as paramount. This consideration is enshrined in the phrase 'personal medical service' as applied to general practice. The ethical duty of the GP towards his patient is clear. Increasingly, this attitude is difficult to sustain; the GP needs to consider each individual patient in the context of the needs and demands of the practice population and society as a whole. The ethical emphasis has shifted somewhat towards a utilitarian viewpoint. It will be important not to lose sight of the individual as the system becomes more complex and responsibilities are distributed among different professionals within the practice. Who is going to decide what is beneficent and what is just? If we consider the general practice team as a whole, as the Tavistock Group has said:

> All those involved in the healthcare system must be committed to developing and applying the specific skills needed to work creatively in the presence of interpersonal and intergroup tensions

and ethical principles will need to be agreed by all those working in the new system.[7]

The future GP

We accept that doctors are made not born; in order to function as a professional in medicine the individual needs to undergo a process of education and training. The attitude and behaviour of the doctor are likely to be formed by this process. At the extreme, we could say that a tightly structured scientific and technical medical education, that concentrates on the acquisition of knowledge and skills, will produce a medical profession peopled by skilled technical scientists.

This denies the concept that the practice of medicine is an art. As long ago as 1978, Pickering said that:

> The doctor's task is to help his patients to live the fullest lives possible ... A narrow education or training is not the best preparation for his life's work ... [H]is material is man, his mind, his body and his place in society.[8]

He was concerned that the medical student's intellectual freedom was intolerably restricted by the 'tyranny' of the system. He feared that the 'straightjacket' of such a system would destroy any creativity, thus inhibiting future development.

Has the system changed since Pickering conducted his survey? We know that postgraduate training for GPs has been developing on very different lines since its introduction in 1967, to the benefit of patients. Will a benefit to patients accrue from the introduction of 'medical humanities' into the medical curriculum? And will a doctor who has been exposed to the humanities at medical school be a 'better' doctor, more understanding of his patients? Already the study of medical ethics is achieving increasing importance in the medical curriculum. Greaves and Evans suggest:

> the gradual emergence of a new viewpoint, in which philosophy and ethics, alongside a whole range of other disciplines, will jointly become reconfigured and so better equipped to address the challenges of contemporary medicine and healthcare.

They would include the discipline of medical humanities as part of this new viewpoint.[9] We will need to see whether the doctor of the future, who has been exposed to the new viewpoint, is also better equipped to address these challenges.

Conclusion

This book is intended to serve as an introduction to a further exploration into the ethical background of the general practitioner's work. Discussion of the different principles that underlie ethical decision making has been brief; nonetheless it indicates the route that may be taken towards acquiring a deeper understanding of the foundation of medical ethics.

References and notes

1   Berlin I (1998) The divorce between the sciences and the humanities. In: *The Proper Study of Mankind*. Chatto and Windus, London, p. 350.
2   By way of illustration, consider Human Rights Act 1998 Article 12 which includes the wording 'right to marry and found a family'. Does this imply a right to successful assisted conception?
3   This is reflected actuarially by the difference in medical indemnity subscriptions between GPs and hospital consultants.
4   Singer P (2000) Medical ethics. *BMJ.* **321**: 283.
5   Sports injuries are often severe and expensive to treat. Private accident insurance is not always in place, as is evidenced by a recent case involving an injury to a player with an amateur football club.
6   Heyd D (1992) *Genethics: moral issues in the creation of people*. University of California Press, London. This text explores the ethics of these issues in more detail.
7   Tavistock Group (1999) A shared statement of ethical principles for those who shape and give health care. *BMJ.* **318**: 249–51.
8   Pickering G (1978) *Quest for Excellence in Medical Education: a personal survey*. Oxford University Press, Oxford.
9   Greaves D and Evans M (2000) Medical humanities (editorial). *J Med Ethics.* **26**: 1–2.

The Hippocratic Oath[1]

I swear by Apollo the physician, and Aesculapius, and Health, and All Heal, and all the gods and goddesses, that, according to my ability and judgement, I will keep this Oath and this stipulation – to reckon him who taught me this Art equally dear to me as parents, to share my substance with him, and to relieve his necessities if required; to look upon his offspring in the same footing as my own brothers, and to teach them this Art, if they shall wish to learn it, without fee or stipulation; and that by precept, lecture and every other mode of instruction, I will impart a knowledge of the Art to my own sons, and those of my teachers, and to disciples bound by a stipulation and oath according to the law of medicine, but to none other.

I will follow that system of regimen which, according to my ability and judgement, I consider for the benefit of my patients, and abstain from whatever is deleterious and mischievous.

I will give no deadly medicine to any one if asked, nor suggest any such counsel; and in like manner I will not give to a woman a pessary to produce abortion.

With purity and holiness I will pass my life and practice my Art. I will not cut persons labouring under the stone, but will leave this to be done by men who are practitioners of this work.

Into whatever houses I enter, I will go into them for the benefit of the sick, and will abstain from every voluntary act of mischief and corruption; and further, from the seduction of females, or males, of freemen or slaves.

Whatever, in connection with my professional practice, or not in connection with it, I see or hear, in the life of men, which ought not to be spoken of abroad, I will not divulge, as reckoning that all such should be kept secret.

While I continue to keep this Oath unviolated, may it be granted to me to enjoy life and the practice of the Art, respected by all men, in all times.

But should I trespass and violate this oath, may the reverse be my lot.

Reference

1 Hippocrates *Works*. Vol. 1: 299–301 (translated by F Adams and NY Loeb).

APPENDIX TWO

A modern Hippocratic Oath

The practice of medicine is a privilege which carries important responsibilities. All doctors should observe the core values of the profession which centre on the duty to help sick people and avoid harm. I promise that my medical knowledge will be used to benefit peoples' health. They are my first concern. I will listen to them and provide the best care I can. I will be honest, respectful and compassionate towards patients. In emergencies I will do my best to help anyone in medical need.

I will make every effort to ensure that the rights of patients are respected including vulnerable groups who lack the means of making their needs known, be it through immaturity, mental incapacity, imprisonment or detention or other circumstance.

My professional judgement will be exercised as independently as possible and not be influenced by political pressures or by factors such as the social standing of the patient. I will not put personal profit or advancement above my duty to patients.

I recognise the special value of human life but I also know that the prolongation of human life is not the only aim of healthcare. Where abortion is permitted, I agree that it should take place only within an ethical and legal framework. I will not provide treatments which are pointless or harmful or which an informed and competent patient refuses.

I will ensure patients receive the information and support they want to make decisions about disease prevention and improvement of their health. I will answer as truthfully as I can and respect patients' decisions unless that puts others at risk of harm. If I cannot agree with their requests I will explain why.

If my patients have limited mental awareness, I will still encourage them to participate in decisions as much as they feel able and willing to do so.

I will do my best to maintain confidentiality about all patients. If there are overriding reasons which prevent my keeping a patient's confidentiality I will explain them.

I will recognise the limits of my knowledge and seek advice from colleagues when necessary. I will acknowledge my mistakes. I will do my best to keep myself and colleagues informed of new developments and ensure that poor standards and practices are exposed to those who can improve them.

I will show respect for all those with whom I work and be ready to share my knowledge by teaching others what I know.

I will use my training and professional standing to improve the community in which I work. I will treat patients equitably and support a fair and humane distribution of health resources. I will try to influence positively authorities whose policies harm public health. I will oppose policies which breach internationally accepted standards of human rights. I will strive to change laws which are contrary to patients' interests or to my professional ethics.

British Medical Association
Annual Report of Council 1996/7

Duties of a doctor[1]

Patients must be able to trust doctors with their lives and well-being. To justify that trust we, as a profession, have a duty to maintain a good standard of practice and care and to show respect for human life. In particular as a doctor you must:

- make the care of your patient your first concern
- treat every patient politely and considerately
- respect patients' dignity and privacy
- listen to patients and respect their views
- give patients information in a way they can understand
- respect the rights of patients to be fully involved in decisions about their care
- keep your professional knowledge and skills up to date
- recognise the limits of your professional competence
- be honest and trustworthy
- respect and protect confidential information
- make sure that your personal beliefs do not prejudice your patients' care
- act quickly to protect patients from risk if you have good reason to believe that you or a colleague may not be fit to practise
- avoid abusing your position as a doctor
- work with colleagues in the ways that best serve patients' interests.

In all these matters you must never discriminate unfairly against your patients or colleagues, and you must always be prepared to justify your actions to them.

Reference

1   Guidance from the General Medical Council in its publication of the same name.

The Human Rights Act 1998

This act establishes in law, from 2 October 2000, the European Convention of Human Rights.

Provisions that are relevant to healthcare are listed below.

Article 1: Dignity of the human person

The dignity of the human person must be respected and protected. Everyone is equal before the law.

Article 2: Right to life

1   Everyone's right to life shall be protected by law. No one shall be deprived of life intentionally save in the execution of a sentence of a court following his conviction of a crime for which this penalty is provided by law.
2   Deprivation of life shall not be regarded as inflicted in contravention of this Article when it results from the use of force which is no more than absolutely necessary:
    (a)   in defence of any person from unlawful violence
    (b)   in order to effect a lawful arrest or to prevent the escape of a person lawfully detained.

Article 3: Prohibition of torture

No one shall be subjected to torture or to inhumane or degrading treatment or punishment.

Article 5: Right to liberty and security

1   Everyone has the right to liberty and security of person. No one shall be deprived of his liberty save in the following cases and in accordance with a procedure prescribed by law:
    (a)   the lawful detention of a person after conviction by a competent court
    (e)   the lawful detention of persons for the prevention of the spreading of infectious diseases, of persons of unsound mind, alcoholics or drug addicts or vagrants.
4   Everyone who is deprived of his liberty by arrest or detention shall be entitled to take proceedings by which the lawfulness of his detention shall be decided speedily by a court and his release ordered if the detention is not lawful.

Article 8: Right to respect for private and family life

1   Everyone has the right to respect for his private and family life, his home and his correspondence.
2   There shall be no interference by a public authority with the exercise of this right except such as is in accordance with the law and is necessary in a democratic society in the interests of national security, public safety or the economic well-being of the country, for the prevention of disorder or crime, for the protection of health or morals, or for the protection of the rights and freedom of others.

Article 9: Freedom of thought, conscience and religion

1   Everyone has the right to freedom of thought, conscience and religion; this right includes freedom to change his religion or belief and freedom, either alone or in community with others

and in public or private, to manifest his religion or belief, in worship, teaching, practice and observance.

2 Freedom to manifest one's religion or beliefs shall be subject only to such limitations as are prescribed by law and are necessary in a democratic society in the interests of public safety, for the protection of public order, health or morals, or for the protection of the rights and freedom of others.

Article 10: Freedom of expression

1 Everyone has the right to freedom of expression. This right shall include freedom to hold opinions and to receive and impart information and ideas without interference by public authority.

Article 12: Right to marry

Men and women of marriageable age have the right to marry and to found a family, according to the national laws governing the exercise of this right.

Article 14: Prohibition of discrimination

The enjoyment of the rights and freedoms set forth in this Convention shall be secured without discrimination on any ground such as sex, race, colour, language, religion, political or other opinion, national or social origin, association with a national minority, property, birth or other status.

Note

Source: *The Human Rights Act 1998*. Schedule 1. Home Office: Guidance for Departments, Annex C.

Glossary[1]

Addiction	Compulsive dependency on a substance that may be obtained legally or illegally. It has the potential to injure health and includes forms of substance abuse, often out of control of the addict. The term is usually perceived as pejorative, and addicts *blamed* for their persistent habit of addiction.
A priori	Reasoning by deduction without the support of valid evidence or experience.
Attitude	A view of something or someone, held by an individual or group, which tends to influence their behaviour. The source of an attitude can be difficult to identify, usually being deep-seated. Because of this, attitudes may be fixed and difficult to alter by logical reasoning.
Autonomy	Freedom to determine one's own actions, the state of self-determination. Linked strongly to Kant's categorical imperative, where a person is an end in himself and never a means to an end.
Belief	What is held to be true – by an individual, a group, a community or a culture.
Beneficence	Doing good.
Blame	Allocate responsibility for some fault or wrong.
Capacity	Ability to do something, e.g. give consent.
Causation	Production of an effect.
Coerce	Compel, perhaps by force, without recognition of individual desires. In ethics, the person who is subjected to coercion may be unaware of the process.

Commodification	The commercialisation of a service. Used to describe the sale of organs or human beings.
Common law	Law developed in the courts by precedent following judicial decisions, rather than by statute.
Competence	The *capacity* to make informed decisions.
Consent	Permission for something to be done, agreement.
Contract	A formal agreement.
Desert	Just reward or punishment.
Distributive justice	Fairness in allocating goods or services.
Duty	Force which binds individuals or organisations to legal or moral obligations.
Empirical	Based on experience rather than theory.
Ergo	Hence.
Ethics	The philosophical study of systems of morality that influence human conduct.
Harm	Injury or damage.
Inter alia	Among other things.
Medical humanities	The study of art, music and literature as an addition to medical education based on the sciences.
Moral	A sense of right and wrong.
Non-maleficence	Doing no harm. Note that it has a link with beneficence, but is not its antonym.
Nosology	Classification of diseases.
Obligation	Legal or moral requirement.
Ontology	The nature of being (philosophical term).
Per se	In itself.
Person	An individual characterised by consciousness, rationality and a moral sense.
Phenomenonology	The study of conscious experience. A term used in psychiatry to describe clinical observations.
Prima facie	At first sight or impression. In ethics often taken to mean a principle is determinative unless overwhelmed by another.
Qua	As, in the capacity of.
Responsibility	Accountability for actions.

Right	A just claim on others, who act as agents responsible for fulfilling the right. Thus there can be no right if there is no agent.
Risk	Probability of an occurrence that may be damaging.
Statutory	Authorised by formal law passed by Parliament.
Value	Worth, intrinsic or perceived.
Will	Ability to make conscious and deliberate choices.

Note

1 Constructed with reference to *Collins English Dictionary* (3e) (1994) HarperCollins, Glasgow.

Further reading

Aristotle (1925) *The Nicomachean Ethics*. Oxford University Press, Oxford.

Beauchamp TL and Childress JF (1994) *Principles of Medical Ethics* (4e). Oxford University Press, Oxford.

Bloch S and Chodoff P (eds) (1991) *Psychiatric Ethics*. Oxford Medical Publications, Oxford.

Brazier M (1992) *Medicine Patients & the Law*. Penguin, Harmondsworth.

Dworkin R (1977) *Taking Rights Seriously*. Duckworth, London.

Dworkin R (1994) *Life's Dominion*. Vintage Books, New York.

Dworkin R (ed.) (1977) *The Philosophy of Law*. Oxford University Press, Oxford.

Gillon R (1995) *Philosophical Medical Ethics*. Wiley, Chichester.

Glover J (1977) *What Sort of People Should There Be?* Penguin, London.

Glover J (ed.) (1990) *Utilitarianism and its Critics*. Macmillan, Basingstoke.

Glover J (1990) *Causing Death and Saving Lives*. Penguin, Harmondsworth.

Hare RM (1997) *Sorting out Ethics*. Oxford University Press, Oxford.

Harris J (1985) *The Value of Life: an introduction to medical ethics*. Routledge, London.

Kant I (1989) *Groundwork of the Metaphysics of Morals* translated by Paton HJ. Routledge, London.

Kennedy I (1988) *Treat Me Right: essays in medical law and ethics*. Oxford University Press, Oxford.

McIntyre A (1981) *After Virtue*. Duckworth, London.

Mason JK and McCall Smith RA (1994) *Law and Medical Ethics* (4e). Butterworths, London.

Mill JS (1962) *Utilitarianism*, M Warnock (ed.). Fontana, London.

Mill JS (1859 reprinted 1975) *3 Essays: on liberty, representative government, and the subjection of women*. Oxford University Press, Oxford.

Montgomery J (1997) *Health Care Law*. Oxford University Press, Oxford.

Newdick C (1995) *Who Should We Treat*. Oxford University Press, Oxford.

Nozick R (1974) *Anarchy, State and Utopia*. Blackwell, Oxford.

Rachels J (1995) *The Elements of Moral Philosophy*. McGraw Hill, New York.

Rawls J (1972) *A Theory of Justice*. Oxford University Press, Oxford.

Singer P (ed.) (1986) *Applied Ethics*. Oxford University Press, Oxford.

Singer P (1993) *Practical Ethics.* Cambridge University Press, Cambridge.

Smart JJC and Williams B (1973) *Utilitarianism: for and against.* Cambridge University Press, Cambridge.

Toon P (1999) *Towards a Philosophy of General Practice: a study of the Virtuous Practitioner.* RCGP Occasional Paper 78.

Index